# Osseointegration in Dentistry: An Introduction

# Osseointegration in Dentistry
## An Introduction

Edited by

**Philip Worthington, MD, BSc, FDSRCS**

University of Washington
Seattle, Washington

**Brien R. Lang, DDS, MS**

University of Michigan
Ann Arbor, Michigan

**William E. LaVelle, DDS, MS**

University of Iowa
Iowa City, Iowa

**Quintessence Publishing Co, Inc**

Chicago, Berlin, London, Tokyo, Moscow,
Prague, São Paolo, Sophia, Warsaw

Library of Congress Cataloging-in-Publication Data

Osseointegration in dentistry: an introduction / edited by Philip
    Worthington, Brien R. Lang, and William E. LaVelle.
        p.    cm.
    Includes bibliographical references.
    ISBN 0-86715-281-8 (soft cover: alk. paper)
    1. Osseointegrated dental implants. I. Worthington, Philip.
II. Lang, Brien R. III. LaVelle, William E.
    [DNLM: 1. Dental Implantation, Endosseous.  WU 640  1994]
RK667.I45086   1994
617.6'9--dc20
DNLM/DLC                                                             94-5464
for Library of Congress                                                 CIP

© 1994 by Quintessence Publishing Co, Inc, Carol Stream, Illinois.
All rights reserved.

Editorial Production: Adam Haus
Cover Design:Jennifer Sabella
Illustration: Allegis, Inc.
Printing and Binding: Ovid Bell Press, Fulton, Missouri

# Contents

# Contributors

**Michael R. Arcuri**
Assistant Professor
Department of Otolaryngology
College of Medicine
University of Iowa
Iowa City, Iowa

**Merle J. Jaarda**
Assistant Professor
Department of Prosthodontics
School of Dentistry
University of Michigan
Ann Arbor, Michigan

**Brien R. Lang**
Professor and Chair
Department of Prosthodontics
School of Dentistry
University of Michigan
Ann Arbor, Michigan

**William E. LaVelle**
Professor
Department of Otolaryngology
College of Medicine
University of Iowa
Iowa City, Iowa

**Michael E. Razzoog**
Associate Professor
Department of Prosthodontics
School of Dentistry
University of Michigan
Ann Arbor, Michigan

**Clark Stanford**
Assistant Professor
Dows Institute of Dental Research
Department of Prosthodontics
University of Iowa
Iowa City, Iowa

**Philip Worthington**
Professor and Chairman
Department of Oral and
Maxillofacial Surgery
School of Dentistry
University of Washington
Seattle, Washington

# Preface

This text is intended to introduce the reader to the concept of osseointegration and its place in modern dental practice. It is a primer, not a technical manual, and it is hoped that it will serve to orient the beginner to the profound impact that osseointegration has had on clinical dentistry.

Basic concepts are presented and the place of osseointegration in the overall scheme of dental treatment planning is illustrated. The reader will come to realize that osseointegration refers not to a development in technique but to a fundamental biological phenomenon with far-reaching applications throughout the fields of medicine and dentistry. Its importance is difficult to overestimate, but most would agree that it is one of the most significant advances in dentistry in the last half century. This book is aimed at dental students who need a simple introduction to the topic while familiarizing themselves with traditional patterns of dental treatment, and at dental practitioners who are beginning to study osseointegration and its applications. For further study, it is anticipated that readers will progress to more advanced texts such as *Tissue Integration Prostheses* (Brånemark, Zarb, and Albrektsson, editors) and *Advanced Osseointegration Surgery* (Worthington and Brånemark, editors).

1

# Introduction

*Philip Worthington*

Since tooth loss from disease and trauma has always been a feature of mankind's existence, it is not surprising that the history of tooth replacement is a long one. Evidence from ancient civilizations shows that attempts were made to replace missing teeth by banding artificial tooth replacements to remaining teeth with metal many centuries ago.

There are two elements in tooth replacement: material for the replacement of teeth, and some form of attachment mechanism. Throughout the ages, and particularly during this century, great ingenuity has been devoted to both these components. Various materials have been used for replacement teeth, including carved ivory and bone. At times, natural teeth extracted from the poor have been used to provide replacements for the missing teeth of the wealthy. In more recent times, porcelain and plastic have provided most of the replacement units.

As for the mechanism of attachment, clinicians have long sought an analog for the periodontal ligament. Experiments were made, sometimes by the unscrupulous on the unsuspecting, in vain attempts to develop a fibrous attachment that could serve the same purposes as the periodontal ligament. The latter is, however, a specialized structure which serves not only as an efficient attachment mechanism but also as a shock absorber and

## History of Implants

a sensory organ. It is furthermore capable of mediating bony remodeling and allowing tooth movement. Easy to underestimate, it is impossible to reproduce. The search for an artificial periodontal ligament has proven fruitless and misguided.

Implants may indeed be anchored in bone by means of a surrounding sheath of connective tissue, but in general this has not shown the degree of organization and specialization that would allow it to pass as a substitute for a periodontal ligament. In most cases, loading leads to gradual widening of the fibrous tissue layer and loosening of the implant, with consequent implant failure. In contrast to the periodontal ligament, a fibrous tissue sheath is a poorly-differentiated layer of scar tissue.

An alternative attachment mechanism was discovered, by means of an accidental finding, during experimental work carried out in Sweden by Professor Per-Ingvar Brånemark and his colleagues during the 1950s and 1960s. Brånemark was a physician—not a dentist—with an interest in the microcirculation of bone and the problems of wound healing. He studied these by means of vital microscopy, a technique whereby a thin layer of living tissue is prepared and examined under the microscope. To facilitate this, he used an implantable optical device, housed in metal and placed surgically into the bone of the experimental animal. This observation chamber allowed light to be transmitted through the thin tissue layer; circulatory and cellular changes could thus be observed in the living tissue. This technique was not new. Similar observation chambers had been used by other researchers. What became significant, however, was that when the metal titanium was used for the observation chamber and the device was introduced into the bone with a gentle surgical technique, the bone was found to adhere to the metal with great tenacity.

The metallic structure became incorporated in the living bone in a way formerly believed to be impossible. Brånemark realized the significance of this new form of attachment mechanism, not merely for dental implant purposes but for orthopedic uses, too, and he called it *osseointegration*. He then set about studying the phenomenon in great detail.

Certain circumstances are necessary for titanium to become rigidly incorporated into living bone. The titanium surface must not be merely clean or even sterile; it must be free from contamination and in a reactive state. The bony implant bed must be prepared with great gentleness, inflicting minimal damage to the tissue. Close congruency of the metallic item and the bone is important. A period of undisturbed healing time is needed to allow the bone to grow up to and fuse with the layer of oxides on the implant surface. If all the desirable circumstances are present, then osseointegration of this unique metal takes place—predictably—in a high percentage of cases.

Prior to the Brånemark era, many ingenious clinicians had worked with many designs of implantable devices intended to support a dental superstructure. These included frameworks resting on the jaw but beneath the mucoperiosteum; frameworks that had bony contact only at the mandibular symphysis and at the ascending rami, but which were otherwise supramucosal; and a wide variety of intraosseous devices of varying shapes and sizes. Some of these could function well over many years, and they kept hope alive for the developing field of implantology. Others failed at varying rates, and tended to gain a bad reputation. In these early implants, predictability was lacking.

The significance of the Brånemark work is that it stressed the need to understand biology, to use the natural healing processes of the body when introducing a metallic foreign body into the bone. The prepared implant site was viewed, correctly, as a wound—a wound in which tissue injury had to be minimized. The special characteristics of titanium were important, particularly its resistance to corrosion and its biocompatibility. It seems that when the necessary conditions are present, living bone has difficulty in recognizing that titanium is a foreign substance.

The successful osseointegrated implant is therefore one in which there is a direct connection between living bone and titanium. This attachment must, and can, endure under conditions of loading. There is no fibrous tissue sheath surrounding the implant; hence the osseointegrated implant is more akin to an ankylosed tooth root than a normal tooth root.

# What is Osseointegration?

Osseointegration is a biological concept. It refers to the incorporation within living bone of an inanimate (metallic) component. It is in essence an anchorage mechanism, nothing more, nothing less. Such anchorage allows the attachment of prosthetic components to the skeleton by means of these anchorage units. The success of osseointegration has been proven beyond all doubt, but achieving successful osseointegration depends on careful planning, meticulous surgical technique, and skillful prosthetic management. It demands an appreciation for biology and an understanding of wound healing in particular. Its applications are wide ranging, including not only dental prostheses but maxillofacial prostheses, replacement of diseased joints and the attachment of artificial limbs. The chapters that follow provide a better understanding of this fascinating biological phenomenon.

# Types of Dental Implants

There are now so many proprietary brands of implants available that it is not feasible to survey them all in this introductory text. The student should be aware, however, of the ways in which dental implants may be classified and must understand the general categories into which they fit. Implants may be classified according to their position, their constituent material, and their morphological design.

### Position

Implants may be *subperiosteal, transosseous,* or *endosseous.*

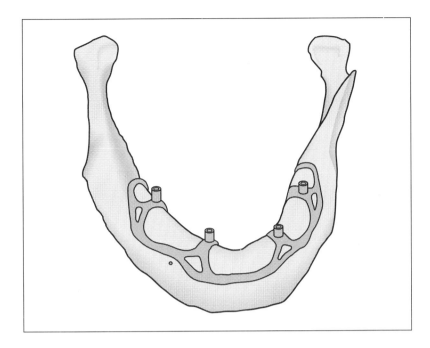

**Fig 1-1**  Subperiosteal implants are custom-cast frameworks supported by the mandible.

## Subperiosteal Implants

This type consists of a nonosseointegrated framework that rests on the surface of the jaw (Fig 1-1). It can be used for either the maxilla or the mandible, although most subperiosteal implants are mandibular. Subperiosteal implants are usually bilateral, but they can be unilateral. The framework rests beneath the mucoperiosteum, with posts that penetrate the mucosa into the mouth, usually supporting an overdenture. Some of these implants have served patients well for many years, but even the best series have shown marked failure rates after 10 years, and many more have lasted much shorter times. Problems have included infection, exteriorization by downgrowth of epithelium, and damage to the underlying bone. Removal may also be difficult.

## Transosseous Implants

The most common form of this implant is the transmandibular staple, which has a plate that fits against the lower border of the mandible at the symphysis and which

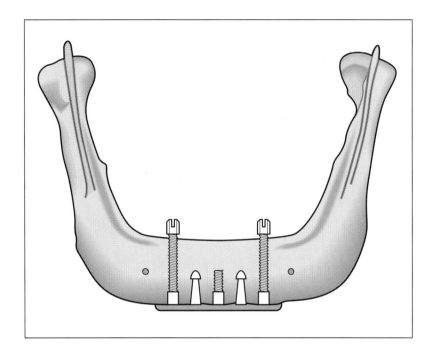

**Fig 1-2**   The mandibular staple bone plate is an exemplary form of transosseous implant.

has posts rising from it (Fig 1-2). Some of these posts pass into the jaw and others pass through it into the mouth, where they serve to stabilize a denture. Some are made of vitallium, some of titanium alloy, and some of gold alloy. Transosseous implants are introduced through a submental incision, usually under general anesthesia in a hospital setting. They are used only for the mandible. Bone loss around the posts has proved a frequent problem.

*Endosseous Implants*

These are placed into the maxilla or mandible through intraoral incisions in the mucoperiosteum (Fig 1-3). The shapes and construction materials vary. Endosseous implants are the most commonly used implant type, and this is the fastest growing part of the dental implant market. They may be used for single tooth replacement, partially edentulous jaws, and totally edentulous jaws. Most claim to be osseointegrated.

## Materials

Many materials have been used for implants, including ceramics such as aluminum oxide and metals ranging from alloys of gold, titanium, and nickel-chrome-vanadium to commercially pure titanium.

## Designs

Many endosseous implants conform more or less to the shape of a tooth root, being either in the form of a tapered cylinder or a true cylinder. Some have threads on the external surface, others do not (Fig 1-3). Some are solid screws. Some have external fins rather than threads. Some are hollow cylinders with fenestrations, called *baskets*. Still others are flat plates, called *blades* (Fig 1-3). Many of these endosseous implants are made of commercially pure titanium or a titanium alloy, and some are finished with a titanium plasma-sprayed surface. Others have a coating of hydroxyapatite, a porous ceramic bone substitute, which may allow the ingrowth of living bone and hence improve anchorage.

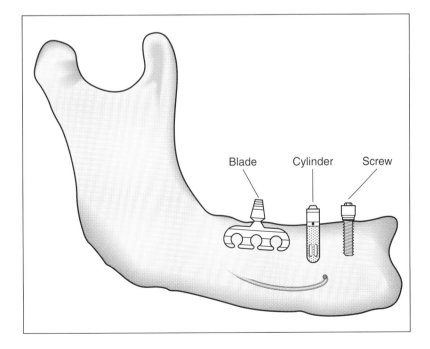

**Fig 1-3**  Endosseous implant designs are varied. Cylinder and screw types are more recent and more successful than blade types.

The clinician may easily be bewildered by the variety of implants available. In making a selection of one or more implant systems for use, it is important to remember to view all manufacturers' claims with healthy skepticism. A survey of practicing dentists provided the following list of features thought important in making a choice of implant system:

- Demonstrated reliability (over at least 5 years)
- American Dental Association approval
- Quality of instrumentation
- Quality of prosthodontics
- Versatility
- Reputation of the manufacturing company
- Ease of use
- Training and after-sales service
- Cost to the patient
- Start-up cost

In evaluating an implant system, the clinician may well ask the following:

- Were animal experiments conducted before the product was marketed?
- Were prospective clinical trial undertaken?
- Are the results of at least 5-year-long trials published in reputable journals?
- Have there been multicenter replication studies?

The practitioner should realize that it is not valid to extrapolate results from one product to another merely on the basis of some superficial morphological resemblance. The composition of the material, its purity, its surface characteristics, and its preparation are of vital importance. Furthermore, the reports of implant trials should state clearly the criteria used for judging success, and studies should report all implants consecutively placed, not merely selected cases.

# 2

# Biocompatibility, Tissue Responses, and the Concept of the Interface

*Clark Stanford*

When biological tissues such as bone and other connective tissues interact with inorganic metals a variety of responses can occur. These reactions can vary from highly reactive processes, which include the formation of corrosion products from metals such as stainless steel, to passive reactions on metals possessing a high reactive surface energy that interacts with oxygen, forming what are known as passivated surface oxides. These oxides form a relatively stable layer on the surface of certain metals when metal ions (M) interact thermodynamically with oxygen, forming stable oxide species ($MO_x$). There are many metals that form surface oxides, such as aluminum, chrome cobalt, nickel chrome. Most of these, however, are not useful as long-term biomaterials because corrosion of the metals causes a continuous release of metallic ions into the surrounding tissues, which may result in significant adverse local and systemic responses. These responses often include both acute and chronic localized inflammatory responses (Type IV) resulting in the eventual encapsulation of the implant in a fibrous capsule, as the body attempts to wall off the offensive material from itself.

Titanium, a common metal, is lightweight, corrosion resistant, and easily milled into useful shapes while retaining its strength. It is often used in ship and air-

## Surface Oxides and Biocompatibility

plane construction because of these properties, which also make it a useful material to use in the human body. Titanium spontaneously forms a tenacious surface coating of titanium oxide (primarily titanium dioxide, $TiO_2$), thus providing a stable ceramic interface on which mineralizing bone matrix can be deposited. This oxide surface provides an initial 50 to 100 Å reactive surface that becomes coated by plasma proteins (especially fibronectin and vitronectin) at the time of implant placement. It is from the biological inertness of this oxide surface that implants derive the important property of biocompatibility. A biocompatible bone-anchored material provides a surface for a cellular and tissue healing response that would occur in a normal undisturbed situation, in situ, if the implant or other artificial material were not present. In essence, this means that an osseointegrated implant's tissue contact is the provisional result of an ongoing bone modeling and remodeling process with a lack of an excessive resorptive response. Therefore, it is important to understand that the integration of bone against the side of an implant is a dynamic process of bone formation and resorption. The balance between these processes is affected by a variety of stimuli, including biomechanical forces delivered through the prosthetic/implant system and the potential presence of peri-implant inflammation.

## Healing Responses

Since the healing response of bone creates the formation of a complex mineralizing matrix, the healing response of the biological tissues and the oxide surface is really a two-phase ceramic interaction between the newly forming hydroxyapatite bone matrix and the surface ceramic oxide. In turn, the thickness, composition, and (potentially) the reactive nature of the implant's ceramic oxide is sensitive to the way in which the surface of the implant is cleaned and sterilized by the manufacturer. In fact, it is postulated that long-term failures of some bone-anchored implants may be due to the presence of minor constituents in the oxide surface (eg, iron) that can interfere with the long-term bone modeling and remodeling processes. The cleaning and handling procedures for implants, which include scrupulous surface cleaning in a controlled environment and minimal handling by the operator prior to the time of placement, are thus of great importance. In addition to the surface contaminants, a number of other physical and chemical features of the oxide layer will influence biological responses to implants. These features include the surface chemistry (oxide composition and thickness), surface energy, and surface topography (size, shape, roughness, etc).

When an implant is placed into a prepared site, the ability of the body to respond to the "trauma" induced by this procedure will influence the kind of tissue response (and hence the degree of integration), even though an implant is composed of a biocompatible material. Proper surgical handling of the tissues with minimal generation of heat (<47°C for 1 minute or less) during preparation of the surgical site will provide the most predictable healing response. Following the formation of an initial clot around the surgical site, a minor inflammatory response occurs which includes the proliferation and differentiation of numerous phagocytes and undifferentiated mesenchymal cells from the adjacent periosteum. The ability of the tissues to differentiate will depend on the presence of an intact vascular bed that provides adequate oxygenation for bone differentiation. Regions where the blood supply has been compromised will lead to an oxygen-poor environment that stimulates the proliferation of fibrous and cartilaginous tissues instead of a mineralizing bone matrix.

Following the initial placement of an implant, a thin (about 0.5 mm) layer of bone in the prepared site will become necrotic (composed of dead and dying cells) simply from the process of forming the implant site. This bone must be replaced by the body as integration proceeds. Initially, an ingrowth of vascular loops will occur at the rate of 0.5 mm per day, followed by initial woven bone formation in the first 2 weeks after initial surgical implant placement. Due to the inert nature of the oxide surface, newly differentiating osteoblastic cells derived from the adjacent periosteum can synthesize a woven bone matrix that provides an initial bone contact with the oxide surface. Following this initial contact, a remodeling phase is initiated, in which hematopoietic-derived osteoclastic cells form cutting cones that will remove the established woven matrix (at a rate of 40 μm per day). Following the resorptive cutting cones, an osteogenic front of lamellar bone differentiation occurs where newly differentiated osteoblasts lay down a mature haversian bone system in a process that is influenced by environmental factors such as micromovements of the interface, local vascular supply, and systemic and local release of matrix-regulating growth factors. In time, the space between the implant and the bone will heal with new bone by a reparative osteogenesis, referred to as creeping substitution, resulting in the clinical fixation of the implant.

The initial healing processes have been studied in optical healing chambers in which a fibrovascular tissue grows into the region of the screw threads (at the phenomenal rate of 85.5 μm per day!), peaking around the third week following implant placement. Under an electron microscope, this growing interface exhibits an ultrastructural relationship involving an intimate contact between the extracellular matrix formed by maturing osteoblastic cells and the titanium oxide surface. Linder and others[1] were able to describe a 20 to 50 nm space between the oxide surface and the nearest collagen fibrils that is filled by complexes of glycosaminoglycans, which probably play a role in mediating adhesion of the mineralizing extracellular matrix to the oxide layer. When transmission electron imaging of the interface from clinically osseointegrated implants was evaluated, areas were described where bone was found to contact the oxide layer directly without an extensive fibrous tissue matrix. Osteoblast-like cells were described to be in close proximity to the interface, separated from the oxide surface by this thin layer of proteoglycan and an amorphous zone (with thicknesses up to 400 nm).

When an implant is placed into the body, the interface between the oxide surface and the bone is not a clearly demarked border, but a region where implant and tissues interactions occur over distances as long as a millimeter or more. Research on pure titanium and titanium alloy (Ti-6Al-4V) orthopedic implants has long suggested that the oxide surface is sensitive to dissolution processes when placed in the body; trace metallic ions can be measured at a distance from the implant itself. Thus, when one is selecting a biomaterial for use, it is important to evaluate the potential harm free ions derived from its composition may have on local and systemic physiological systems. Observation of a clinically loaded dental implant by Hanawa[2] revealed a fascinating series of changes. Six years after placement, a passivated titanium oxide layer of 2,000Å was observed. When the composition of the newly formed oxide was evaluated, it was found to contain organic and inorganic (Ca, P, and S) materials, suggesting that the implant's surface oxide was reactive and sensitive to growth and uptake of mineral ions, even though it was coated with a protein layer. When pure titanium or titanium alloy (Ti-6Al-4V) surfaces are exposed to physiological blood, as occurs at the time of implantation, complex titanium-phosphate and calcium-containing hydroxyl groups spontaneously form on the oxide surface, indicating that titanium reacts with water, mineral ions, and plasma fluids. Interestingly, the low pH (pH = 5.2) found in the recipient implant bed may actually accelerate the formation of calcium phosphate mineral on the surface of the pure titanium surface.[2] Recent work by numerous investigators has demonstrated a measurable release of titanium ions (and aluminum, in the case of titanium alloy) into the tissues surrounding implants once they are in place. The oxide surface is therefore a dynamic system, not passive in nature. The oxide surface plays a role, along with bone remodeling, in creating an adaptive interfacial region rather than simply a sharply demarcated boundary between the implant and the body. Thus, the reactive nature of this oxide surface, with its spontaneous formation of a calcium-phosphate apatite, is one reason why titanium appears to be so biocompatible. It is truly

# The Dynamic Oxide Interface

unusual that an inorganic material will coat itself and thus literally present itself to the body with a physiological disguise.

Although osseointegrated implants can appear to be stable from a clinical point of view, it is important to remember that the biological response to the oxide surface is dynamic and constantly changing. A common method to evaluate biological responses of healing to an implant is to evaluate the extent of bone contact that can be measured in the microscope at the light level (referred to as histomorphometry). In evaluating the "integrated" state of an implant, this degree of contact is compared to the relative strength that the implant has when one attempts to remove it. While it is unclear at the present time how much bone contact is needed for a long-term clinically stable implant, it does appear consistent that the following is true. When the amount of bony contact is evaluated around an implant, the degree of trabecular contact will vary between 30% and 70%, with a mean around 50% contact. The amount of contact can vary significantly, depending on where the measurement is made on any one implant, and the degree of bone contact will change with progressive bone remodeling. This latter concept can be termed *progressive osseointegration.*

## Progressive Osseointegration

"Osseointegration" implies a dynamic interface environment (Fig 2-1) that will become more mature with the proper loading of the implant, following an initial healing phase in which the neonatal healing site is not subjected to any stress or micromotion (displacement of the implant relative to the bone). Premature micromotion will repeatedly disrupt the normal osseous modeling processes, leading to the formation of a fibrous scar tissue around the implant. Once the initial osseous fixation is allowed to occur, abutments are then connected and a careful and precise regimen of progressive loading of the implants must be developed. This need for progressive loading is due to the nature of the interface region. It is well known in orthopedics that for proper bone develop-

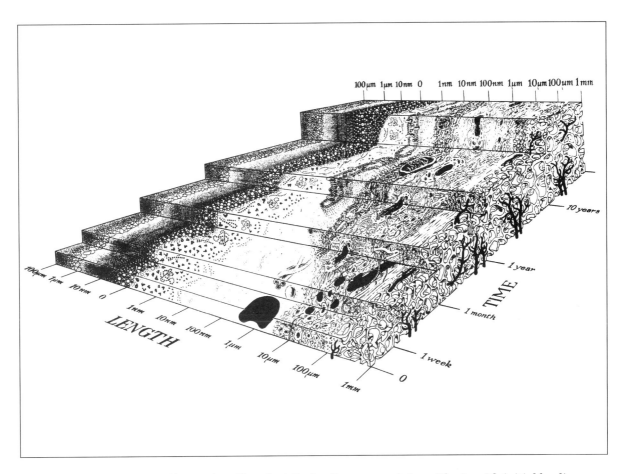

**Fig 2-1**   Progressive osseointegration. Note that the healing process is logarithmic, with initial healing occurring in the first month, followed by tissue maturation through the first year after placement. Notice how the oxide layer is reactive and grows as remodeling of the osseous bed leads to enhanced tissue integration. The inset shows the general distribution of layers, as well as how connective tissue formation may occur, resulting in fibrous encapsulation and incomplete integration. (Reprinted with permission from Kasemo and Lausmaa, Surface science aspects on inorganic biomaterials. CRC Crit Rev Biocompatibility 1986; 2:335–380.)

ment and maintenance a certain level of mechanical strain (typically 1,000 μ-strain) is needed in a cyclical pattern on a daily basis. It is the response of bone to the applied mechanical forces which influences the modeling and remodeling processes in order to maintain homeostasis. It is thus interesting that once initial healing is allowed to occur in dental implants, the degree of bone contact increases from 53% to 74% by the end of the first year following insertion[3] when the implants are loaded in a proper manner. In the region of the transcortical passage this can eventually amount to over 90% bone contact.[4] When the implant interface is monitored radiographically, an increase in the osseous trabecula in the region around the implants is often described in the first few years following placement; a feature which suggests that the body's normal remodeling responses are adapting to the physiological loading of the implant-supported prosthesis.

In addition to the surface chemistry, the physical properties of an implant surface influence the integrated implant's retentive strength. A titanium surface that has been roughened by sandblasting will have significantly higher level of bone contact than titanium surfaces that are polished smooth (50% versus 20%), correlating with greater pullout strengths.[5] When the implant surface is prepared, it is important to create a retentive system that provides for immediate fixation of the implant at the time of placement. This can be achieved by the use of macroretentive features like screw threads or through use of a "press-fit" design, which utilizes a prepared recipient site that is smaller than the implant diameter. It is through use of these macroretentive features that initial micromotion can be prevented. These features also provide a titanium-oxide interface with a larger surface area for integration. The ability to osseointegrate metallic implants is dependent on a combination of proper surgical technique, a metal surface that is biocompatible with the body, and physical features that provide for immediate fixation and stability of the interface region. Successful osseointegration can only be accomplished in a predictable manner by a combination of delicate tissue handling, precise surface science, progressive loading, and a scientific knowledge of the underpinnings which support this tremendous treatment modality.

# References

1.  Linder L, Albrektsson T, Brånemark P-I, Hansson HA, Ivarsson B, Jonsson U, et al. Electron microscopic analysis of the bone-titanium interface. Acta Orthop Scand 1983;54:45–52.

2.  Hanawa T. Titanium and its oxide film: A substrate for formation of apatite. In: Davies JE (ed). The Bone-Biomaterial Interface. Toronto: Univ of Toronto Press, 1991:49–61.

3.  Gottlander M, Albrektsson T. Histomorphometric studies of hydroxylapatite-coated and uncoated CP titanium threaded implants in bone. Int J Oral Maxillofac Implants 1991;6;399–404.

4.  Johansson C, Albrektsson T. Integration of screw implants in the rabbit: a 1-year follow-up of removal torque of titanium implants. Int J Oral Maxillofac Implants 1987;2:69–75.

5.  Buser D, Schenk RK, Steinemann S, Fiorellini JP, Fox CH, Stich H. Influence of surface characteristics on bone integration of titanium implants. A histomorphometric study in miniature pigs. J Biomed Mater Res 1991;25:889–902.

# 3

# Surface Preparation

*Merle J. Jaarda*

There are a number of biological considerations that determine the development of the interface between the host tissues and the implant and influence the lifetime survival rate of dental implants. On the implant side of the interface, the surface preparation of the implant, including bioactive coatings and the formation of titanium oxides, is a significant factor in osseointegration. Transmission of forces from the functioning prosthesis to the surface of the implant, and through to the bone bearing the functional load, is equally important. In the host tissues, the use of bone morphogenetic (inductive) proteins and bone growth factors can promote the process of osseogenesis.

The surface preparation for any implant system involves not only the material used in its fabrication, but the surface composition of the bulk material as well, and any ceramic coatings that may have been applied to this surface.[1] All of these elements must work together to facilitate successful osseointegration.

## Materials

Commercially pure titanium, titanium-aluminum-vanadium (Ti-6Al-4V) alloy, and the ceramic hydroxyapatite are currently the major materials used in endosseous implants in North America.[1] In some implant systems, the dense metallic substrates are modified to create porous surfaces using powder spheres,[2] fibers,[3] or plasma-sprayed coatings.[4] This surface modification is thought to enhance the bond between the bone and the implant surface.

Titanium is the ninth most abundant element on earth, and in its natural state is found as the compound titanium dioxide ($TiO_2$), which is soft yet strong for its weight, and quite ductile. Ti-6Al-4V was alloyed to create a biocompatible material with added strength. The commercially pure titanium recommended for dental implants has a composition of 99.75% titanium, 0.05% iron, 0.1% oxygen, 0.03% nitrogen, 0.05% carbon, and 0.012% hydrogen.[5,6] Both commercially pure titanium and Ti-6Al-4V have excellent corrosion resistance.

Ceramic materials such as hydroxyapatite were selected for use in implant fabrication because of their presumed inertness.[1]

# Surface Composition

The bulk material used to create the implant provides the general characteristics of its composition and biocompatibility; however, surface composition plays the major role in tissue acceptance and osseointegration. Researchers have found that the outer few nanometers of the implant surface exhibit a variable composition that is influenced by the process of fabrication, the methods of cleaning and sterilizing the surface, and the handling during manufacturing and packaging of the implant.[1]

Exposure of the titanium surface to air results in the formation of an initial oxide layer of about 1.0 nm.[7] Varying oxide thicknesses from 3 to 20 nm have been reported on the surface of implants as a result of the methods used in cleaning and sterilizing the implant.[8,9,10]

The oxide layer is considered to be an integral part of the implant, and the depth and composition of the layer may have profound effects on the osseointegration process. However, the optimum thickness or composition of the oxide layer is yet unknown. The most common oxide layer is $TiO_2$, with the other oxides $TiO$ and $Ti_2O_3$ also found on the surface of implants.[8] At body pH, the stable form of the titanium oxide is $TiO_2$, and very little reaction occurs between the body fluids and the titanium in the presence of this oxide.[11]

Some investigators have suggested that the oxide layer may have a controlling influence over the thickness of the collagen-free proteinaceous film found between the implant and the adjacent bone surface. With a commercially pure titanium implant, a proteinaceous film of approximately 20 nm has been reported, while the alloyed titanium Ti-6Al-4V implant, which may have a different oxide layer, produced a 500 nm proteinaceous film.[6]

As previously stated in Chapter 2, the roughness of the titanium surface may affect the bonding of the biological molecules of the host tissues to it. However, there is a lack of agreement among researchers and clinicians regarding the occurrence of such a mechanism. Baier et al[12] have reported that a surface roughness at the level of 1.0 μm and less was not a significant influence on the outcome of the interaction between the implant and the host tissues.

A number of elements in addition to titanium have been found on the implant surface following fabrication, including phosphorus, carbon, calcium, oxygen, silicon, and chlorine.[13] Removal of the contaminating elements and achievement of a perfectly clean implant surface are the goals of the recommended cleaning and sterilization techniques. Suggested techniques are autoclave sterilization, heat sterilization, ultraviolet sterilization, and radiofrequency glow discharge (RFGD) sterilization. All of these methods have been examined in a number of studies; however, the results have been varied. Regardless of the implant preparation technique selected, the surface of any titanium or titanium-alloy implant must be rendered free of contaminants and be in a sterile condition prior to surgical implantation. Improper surface preparation may add to the contamination that may be present, and would certainly adversely affect osseointegration.

## Ceramic Coatings

A variety of studies have suggested that coating of the surface of the implant with bioactive ceramic materials will enhance the bonding of the implant to bone. The most commonly used coating is hydroxyapatite. Numerous published reports show conflicting results regarding the influence of the coatings on the interface; thus, there appears to be a lack of agreement on the use of coatings.[1]

## References

1. Smith DC. Dental implants: Materials and design considerations. Int J Prosthodont 1993;6:106–117.

2. Galante J, Rostoker W, Lueck R, Ray RD. Sintered fiber metal composites as a basis for attachment of implants to bone. J Bone Joint Surg 1971;55A:101–114.

3. Welsh RP, Pilliar RM, Macnab I. Surgical implants: The role of surface porosity in fixation to bone and acrylic. J Bone Joint Surg 1971;55A:963–977.

4. Luthy H, Strub JR, Scharer P. Analysis of plasma flame-sprayed coatings on endosseous oral titanium implants exfoliated in man: Preliminary results. Int J Oral Maxillofac Implants 1987;2:197–202.

5. Albrektsson T, Brånemark P-I, Hansson HA, Kasemo B, Larsson K, Lundström I et al. The interface zone of inorganic implants in vivo: Titanium implants in bone. Ann Biomed Eng 1983;11:1–27.

6. Albrektsson T, Jacobsson M. Bone-metal interface in osseointegration. J Prosthet Dent 1987;57:597–607.

7. Kasemo B, Lausmaa J. Surface science aspects on inorganic biomaterials. Crit Rev Biocompatibility 1986;3:247–259.

8. Brånemark P-I. Introduction to osseointegration. In: Brånemark P-I, Zarb GA, Albrektsson T (eds). Tissue-Integrated Prostheses: Osseointegration in Clinical Dentistry. Chicago: Quintessence, 1985:11–76.

9. Klauber C, Lenz LJ, Henry PJ. Oxide thickness and surface contamination of six endosseous dental implants determined by electron spectroscopy for chemical analysis: A preliminary report. Int J Oral Maxillofac Implants 1990;5:264–271.

10. Keller J, Draughn R, Wightman J, Dougherty W, Meletiou S. Characterization of sterilized CP titanium implant surfaces. Int J Oral Maxillofac Implants 1990;5:360–367.

11.  Lemons J. Dental implant interfaces as influenced by biomaterial and biomechanical properties. In: McKinney RV, Lemons JE (eds). The Dental Implant. Littleton, CO: PSG, 1985:143–152.

12.  Baier RE, Meenaghan MA, Hartman LC, Flynn HE, Natiella JR. Implant surface characteristics and tissue interaction. J Oral Implantol 1988;13:594–606.

13.  Hartman LC, Meenaghan MA, Schaaf NG, Hawker PB. Effects of pretreatment sterilization and cleaning methods on materials properties and osseoinductivity of a threaded implant. Int J Oral Maxillofac Implants 1989;4:11–18.

# 4

# Biomechanics

*Merle J. Jaarda*

Investigators have studied the interface between the implant and the adjacent bone and soft tissues in order to better understand the mechanism of the biological attachment at this important junction. Our body of knowledge has grown extensively, particularly at the cellular and histochemical levels, and the dynamics of this interface have been clearly demonstrated. It is also apparent that the implant side of the interface is equally dynamic, and it is only recently that the role of the implant, especially from a biomechanical perspective, has become the focus of researchers.

Research highlighting biomechanics and implants has come about because investigators and clinicians alike have recognized the importance of the entire implant system in treatment and in the lifetime survival rate of the implants. The variety of prosthodontic hardware used to meet both routine and special rehabilitation needs has increased tremendously since the 1980s. There seems to be a component available for every condition indicating implant use, yet there is little known about the biomechanical influence of the implants themselves on the bone that supports them.

To better understand implant dynamics and their influence on the implant-to-bone interface, it is helpful to consider the implant hardware as a complex consisting of multiple parts. A typical implant complex consists of nine components (Fig 4-1) that are united and function as an integrated unit. The components are:

1. the osseous tissue surrounding the implant,
2. the implant,
3. the abutment (core),
4. the abutment screw (post),
5. the prosthetic coping,
6. the prosthetic retaining screw,
7. the prosthetic framework,
8. the esthetic veneer, and
9. the masticatory surface.

In reality, an interface exists between each of the nine components across which functional loads are transferred and ultimately transmitted to the supporting bone. These nine force transfer sites are called the *prosthodontic interfaces,* and each plays a significant role in the dynamic state of the biomechanics related to the implant.

Studies have been conducted that deal with the following biomechanical areas:

a. the design of implants and their surface characteristics,
b. the shock absorption capabilities of selected implant designs,
c. the stress and strength considerations of abutment and prosthetic retaining screws and
d. the forces that act on the implant prosthesis and that are transmitted to other implant components.

Although the scientific information available on these biomechanical areas and the prosthodontic interfaces is limited, we will consider each in detail.

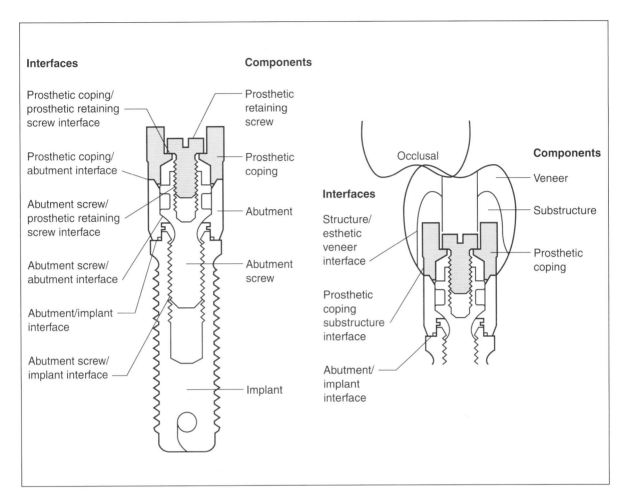

**Fig 4-1** The implant complex, showing the nine components and interfaces.

There is an apparent lack of consensus among researchers regarding the basic design of an implant, as evidenced by the multiplicity of implant designs. Some state that it is critical to load the bone in compression while minimizing the shear forces; the screw-type implants reflect this theory. On the other hand, proponents of cylindrical designs stress the importance of the implant deriving its support through shear forces applied to the implant-to-bone interface; the cylindrical press-fit implants reflect this theory.

# Implant Designs And Surface Characteristics

As previously noted, the surface roughness of an implant's surface has been reported as a biomechanical factor requiring a higher removal torque than a smooth surface.[1]

The *finite element method* (FEM) has been used extensively as a research tool to demonstrate that different implant shapes lead to significant variations in stress distribution in bone. The finite element method uses a two- or three-dimensional computerized mathematical model of the implant-bone complex. The computerized model is dimensionally, mechanically, and physiologically correct. Each component in the implant-bone complex is separated into small fundamental parts called *elements*, which are described as *finite* because the area of each component is predetermined by its shape and size. Different implant shapes have shown significant variations in stress distribution in the adjacent bone using FEM.[2] The smooth-cylinder and screw implant shapes have more uniform stress distribution than the conical or step-shaped implants. A larger-diameter implant has been shown by FEM to produce a more favorable stress distribution at the implant-bone interface.[3] For example, the ultimate pullout force of an implant in dog alveolar bone was shown to strongly correlate with implant length, but not with diameter.[4]

## Shock Absorption

It has been suggested by some investigators that some form of shock absorption is necessary between the implant-abutment and abutment-prosthesis interfaces to cope with the range of forces transmitted from the masticatory surfaces to the supporting bone during mastication. However, scientific evidence to support this theory is very limited. The occlusal forces on implant-supported prostheses appear to be reduced with an internal shock absorber.[5] However, a comparison of the stress-transfer characteristics of a dental implant with rigid or resilient internal elements showed no difference in the deflection of a cantilever beam.[6]

Research on implant screws has involved primarily two areas: the ultimate failure strength of the various screws, and the preload torque (clamping force) applied to these screws (Fig 4-2). This research has been stimulated by two factors: *(1)* the introduction of an increasing number of similarly-designed implant components[7] based on the system originally developed by P.-I. Brånemark, and *(2)* by the recent introduction of torque wrenches that help the clinician uniformly join the implant components to more evenly distribute the forces.[8] Manual tightening of screws can be inconsistent, while mechanical torque-applying devices insure uniform tightening.[9] However, the optimum torque is still controversial, and the theoretical recommendations do not tend to agree with in vitro research reports. The recommendation of a 10-Ncm preload to unite a prosthesis framework or single tooth component to the abutment using the appropriate screw is based on the theory that this 10-Ncm preload is just below the yield strength (the point at which permanent deformation increases rapidly without a corresonding increase in applied load) of the retaining screw and therefore will not cause it to break.[10] However, in vitro research findings have suggested that the optimum preload may be higher.[11] Both the theoretical and in vitro research agree that the optimum preload for a given type of screw should be correlated with the mechanical properties of the specific screw.

# Implant Screws

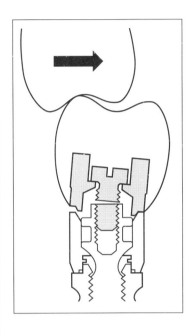

**Fig 4-2**   An implant complex with a fractured prosthetic retaining screw, caused by exceeding the mechanical limits of the screw.

# Implant Prosthesis and Forces

The biomechanics of the implant prosthesis and forces generated by various oral functions have been reported using theoretical models and computer simulations which primarily examine the geometry of this complicated arrangement of dental hardware and its effects on the implant-bone interface. These methods have provided information about both the number of implants in an edentulous arch (a jaw without any teeth), and the importance of positioning the implants in a curved arrangement around the arch, instead of in a flattened

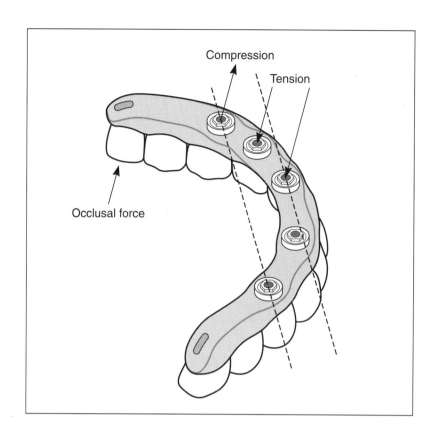

**Fig 4-3a**   A totally edentulous arch with an appropriate number of properly positioned implants to compensate for the load of a fixed implant-supported prosthesis.

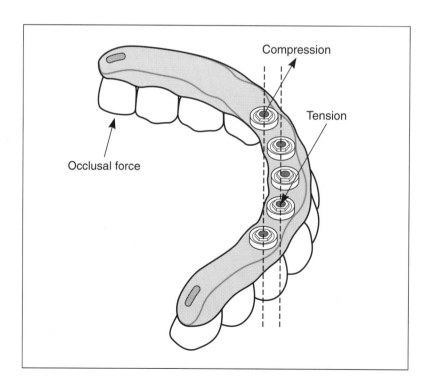

**Fig 4-3b**   A totally edentulous arch with implants positioned along a straight line. This arrangement provides limited compensation for the load of the prosthesis.

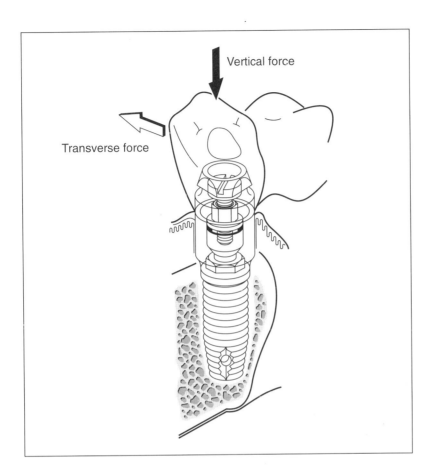

Vertical force

Transverse force

**Fig 4-4** Vertical and transverse forces acting on an implant prosthesis. These forces usually act in combination.

configuration (Figs 4-3a and b), thereby distributing more efficiently the functional forces transferred by the prosthetic framework designs to the implants and bone.[12–16]

Occlusal loading of the implants has also received considerable attention. It has been reported that if the load is applied directly over the implant it is a compressive force, while loads in all other force applications are bending moments of forces (Fig 4-4). In those force applications where bending moments occur, the implant nearest the applied load will still experience a compressive force, and the more distant implants and their related components are placed in tension (Fig 4-5).[16]

New information is continually being introduced by researchers and clinicians regarding these forces and their effects on implant performance at the prosthodontic

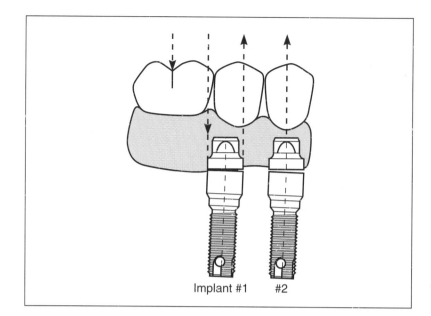

**Fig 4-5**  A bending moment around implant 1 produces a compressive load on the distal edge of this prosthesis. A tensile stress develops on the mesial edge of implant 1 and on all of implant 2.

interfaces. The following factors, by themselves and in various combinations, create extremely complex problems in analysis because of their numbers and the potential for interactions.

- the magnitude, direction, and location of the loading
- the geometry and mechanical properties of the prosthesis framework
- the nature (accuracy and precision of fit) of the component connections
- the number, locations, and angulations of the implants
- the mechanical properties of all the materials involved in the prosthesis construction
- the mechanical properties of the bone and supporting tissues that come in contact with the implant

As one can see, a great deal is yet to be learned about this important area of biomechanics.

Osseointegration of implants in cortical bone is predictable; however, problems will still occur when there is a lack of cortical bone present in the site selected for implant placement. This is especially true in the maxilla, where the cortical plates are extremely thin. It would be ideal if the bone could be stimulated to form a cortical plate around an implant similar to the lamina dura that is seen around natural teeth.

Clinically, it has been reported that placing demineralized bone in the healing wound site results in localized bone formation. In these situations, the bone matrix serves as a storehouse of growth factors, of which transforming growth factor-ß (TGF-ß) has the potential to influence local bone growth. TGF-ß is the prototype of a large family of structurally related regulatory peptides shown to modulate bone remodeling through osteoblastic and osteoclastic activity. TGF-ß has been purified from multiple sources but the largest source of TGF-ß in humans is bone. Recently osseoinductive bone proteins, such as osteogenin, have been isolated. These bone morphogenic proteins are members of the TGF-ß superfamily and have been shown to induce new bone formation, while the other growth factors promote bone growth.[17]

The potential for TGF-ß and other growth factors, such as a platelet-derived growth factor (PDGF), to assist in osseointegration and host acceptance of implants suggests almost limitless opportunities for future research. Initial research reports have demonstrated the ability of these materials to induce and promote bone formation.[18] The potential to coat alloplastic implants with these growth factors may allow the clinician the opportunity to place implants in areas where the quality of the existing bone would normally prohibit implant placement.

Bovine osteogenin has been placed in experimentally created calvarial defects in baboons and has demonstrated significantly more bone regeneration in the wound site of the treated population than in the untreated controls.[19] This same protein, when combined with type I collagen, resulted in greater bone formation in nonhealing calvaria defects in rats.[20] When this protein was combined with hydroxyapatite, the results were

# Bone Substitutes

not as promising, suggesting that the collagen may potentiate the effect of osteogenin by providing a more permissive surface for cell attachment than the hydroxyapatite. Ungrafted controls in this previous study healed with a fibrous connective tissue and a small amount of bone at the periphery.

PDGF-ß and an insulin-like growth factor (IGF-I) in combination have been shown to promote periosteal thickening and bone formation in long bones in adult Yucatan micropigs.[21] Recently, it has been shown that membranous bone contains greater amounts of IGF-II and TGF-ß than does endochondral bone.[22] It is theorized that the increase in these growth factors may explain the clinically seen improved survival rate of membranous grafts over endochondral grafts. The many potentials for these growth factors and for their application to healing implants and osseointegration will continue to be explored.

# References

1.  Carlsson L, Albrektsson B. Removal torques for polished and rough titanium implants. Int J Oral Maxillofac Implants 1988;3:21–24.

2.  Siegel D, Soltesz U. Numerical investigations of the influence of implant shape on the stress distribution in the jaw bone. Int J Oral Maxillofac Implants 1989;4:333–339.

3.  Matsushita Y, Kitoh M, Mizuta K, Ikeda H, Suetsugu T. Two-dimensional FEM analysis of hydroxyapatite implants: Diameter effects on stress distribution. J Oral Implantol 1990;16:6–11.

4.  Block MS, Delgado A and Fontenot MG. The effect of diameter and length of hydroxylapatite-coated dental implants on ultimate pull-out force in dog alveolar bone. J Oral Maxillofac Surg 1990;48:174–178.

5.  Chapman RJ, Kirsch A. Variations in occlusal forces with a resilient internal implant shock absorber. Int J Oral Maxillofac Implants 1990;5:369–374.

6.  McGlumphy EA, Campagni WV, Peterson LJ. A comparison of the stress transfer characteristics of a dental implant with a rigid or a resilient internal element. J Prosthet Dent 1989;62:586–593.

7. Lang BR, McGlumphy E, Lewis S, Christensen GJ. What scientific proof does the restorative clinician have that intersystem implant hardware components are interchangeable without potential harm to long-term survival? (Current Issues Forum) Int J Oral Maxillofac Implants 1993;8:105–115.

8. Nobelpharma Product Catalog. Gothenburg, Sweden: Nobel Industries, 1991:26.

9. Jaarda MJ, Razzoog ME, Gratton DG. Providing optimum torque to implant prostheses: A pilot study. Implant Dent 1993;2:50–52.

10. Rangert B, Jemt T, Jorneus L. Forces and moments on Brånemark implants. Int J Oral Maxillofac Implants 1989;4:241–247.

11. McGlumphy EA, Elfers CL, Mendal DA. A comparison of torsional ductile fracture in implant coronal screws [abstract 72]. J Dent Res 1992;71 (special issue).

12. Brunski JB. Biomechanical considerations in dental implant design. Int J Oral Implant 1988;5:31–34.

13. Skalak R. Aspects of biomechanical considerations. In: Brånemark PI, Zarb GA, Albrektsson T (eds). Tissue-Integrated Prostheses: Osseointegration in Clinical Dentistry. Chicago: Quintessence, 1985:117–128.

14. Brunski JB, Skalak R. Biomechanical considerations. In: Worthington P, Brånemark P-I (eds). Advanced Osseointegration Surgery: Applications In The Maxillofacial Region. Chicago: Quintessence, 1992:15–39.

15. Brunski JB. Forces on dental implants and interfacial stress transfer. In: Laney WR, Tolman DE (eds). Tissue Integration in Oral, Orthopedic, and Maxillofacial Reconstruction. Chicago: Quintessence, 1992:108–124.

16. Rangert B, Gunne J, Sullivan DY. Mechanical aspects of a Brånemark implant connected to a natural tooth: An in vitro study. Int J Oral Maxillofac Implants 1991;6:177–186.

17. Ripamonti U, Reddi AH. Growth and morphogenic factors in bone induction: role of osteogenin and related bone morphogenic proteins in craniofacial and periodontal bone repair. Crit Rev Oral Biol Med 1992;3:1–14.

18. Reddi AH, Cunningham NS. Bone induction by osteogenin and bone morphogenetic proteins. Biomat 1990;11:33–34.

19. Hollinger J, Mark DE, Bach DE, Reddi AH, Seyfer AE. Calvarial bone regeneration using osteogenin. J Oral Maxillofac Surg 1989;47:1182–1186.

20. Doll BA, Towle HJ, Hollinger JO, Reddi AH, Mellonig JT. The osteogenic potential of two composite graft systems using osteogenin. J Periodontol 1990 61:745–750.

21 Lynch SE, Hernandez R, Trippel S, Fox CH, Antoniades HN. Effects of PDGF-ß and IGF-I on bone regeneration [abstract 82]. J Dent Res 1992;71:116.

22. Finkelman RD, Hardesty R, Rakijan D, Eason AL, Abraham SM, Tutundzhyan Y et al. Increased IGF-II and TGB-ß in calvarial bone: Graft survival implications [abstract 83]. J Dent Res 1992;71:116.

# 5

# Intraoral Implant Applications

*Michael E. Razzoog*

The limited success experienced by implant patients during the 1950s and early 1960s left most dentists skeptical about the routine clinical application of implants. Most implants were unpredictable and eventually failed, with some failing more rapidly than others. During the past 25 years, skepticism has been replaced by renewed interest among both specialists and general dentists, due largely to the efforts of P.-I. Brånemark and his coworkers in Sweden, who introduced the concept of osseointegration.[1] In the mid-1960s, Brånemark demonstrated that implants could survive with certainty in the oral environment as long as specific biological principles were not violated. When the principles of osseointegration are followed, the anchorage of a nonbiological titanium implant unit to bone with a direct structural and functional connection between living bone and the surface of a load-carrying implant will occur, with approximately 95% and 85% implant survival rates for maxillae and for mandibles, respectively.[2] Several longitudinal studies of implants placed in edentulous jaws have been conducted to validate osseointegration, and the method has withstood this scientific scrutiny.[3–5]

The scientific breakthrough provided by osseointegration in the past several decades has resulted in implants being fully embraced as a treatment method. There is currently much demographic evidence that implants will become a major service of dentistry during the 1990s and beyond into the 21st century.

Diversity in treatment applications using implants is just beginning to be realized by health care providers. Intraoral implants have been used primarily as replacements for tooth roots, or tooth-root analogs (Fig 5-1). However, implants are not limited to these applications. Implants have also been used with equal success as anchorage to facilitate orthodontic tooth movement, prosthetic treatment of craniofacial defects, and prosthetic joint replacements in the human skeleton. Implants have been used with various bone grafting techniques to improve the bony support of the jaws for dentures. An entirely new approach to the buildup of new bone tissue, called bone apposition, has been formulated using implants in a technique called guided tissue regeneration. Clinicians have also begun to place implants immediately following tooth extraction, rather than waiting until a later time, which has also expanded the opportunities for implant use.

## Increased Need for Dental Implants

Specifically relevant to the clinical applications of implants is the pattern of missing teeth evident from the 1985–86 National Institute for Dental Research national survey of tooth loss and accumulated prosthetic treatment potential in US employed adults and seniors.[6] The data show that in the year 1986 only 10% of 65- to 69-year-olds, 26% of 55- to 64-year-olds, 32% of 45- to 54-year-olds, and 50% of 35- to 44-year olds had no indications for prosthodontic services. Most of the US population over age 35 demonstrated patterns of missing teeth that are clinically consistent with the need for implants.

A conservative estimate suggests a 38% increase in need for prosthodontic services today compared to the need of 25 years ago. The projected unmet need for prosthodontic treatment by 2000 shows that the clinical indications for implant services will expand far into the future.

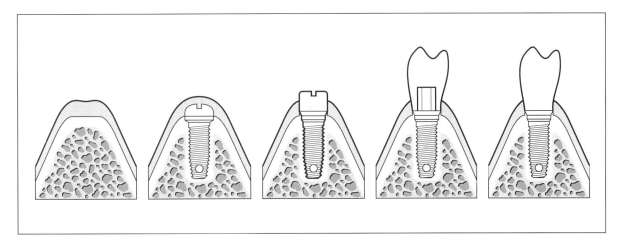

**Fig 5-1** Basic process of single-tooth replacement using an endosseous screw-type implant. From left: the preoperative ridge; initial implant placement with cover screw; abutment placement; initial prosthesis placement; final crown restoration.

Chester Douglass has reported that although the number of people over age 65 may increase from 27 million to 64 million in 2030, the percentage of edentulous persons (currently 33%) is projected to decrease to as low as 15% by the same year.[7] However, the actual number of people needing complete dentures would remain roughly constant at approximately 9 million. By comparison, the numbers of patients in this age category who will be partially edentulous should substantially increase.

It has been estimated that currently 41% of the people over age 40 have edentulous spaces. Given the anticipated increase in the size of the population in need of prosthodontic services by 2000, the clinical applications for implants in partial edentulous areas should grow at an equal rate.

The range of intraoral clinical applications involving dental implants is expanding. Innovative clinicians continue to explore new situations in which implants, as the primary treatment method, can help provide comfortable, functional, and esthetically pleasing solutions to dental problems. There is also increasing use of implants as an alternative to conventional prosthodontic procedures. The intraoral clinical applications of dental implants include the following:

a. treatment of the totally edentulous maxilla and mandible,
b. restoration of anterior and posterior edentulous spaces previously occupied by more than one tooth, which may or may not be bounded by natural teeth, and
c. replacement of the single tooth.

## The Totally Edentulous Arch

The pioneering work in osseointegration has highlighted implants as a pre-prosthetic surgical procedure used to aid totally edentulous patients who have lost excessive amounts of their residual ridges due to bone resorption (reduction of the volume and size of the maxilla and/or mandible) and whose dentures are loose (Fig 5-2). This treatment approach is much more common in the mandibular arch; however, it has also been used successfully in those patients who have lost considerable bone from the anterior maxilla, or whose posterior hard palate creates an acute angle with the soft palate, making denture retention extremely problematic. Both prospective and retrospective studies have underscored the predictability and versatility of osseointegration in large numbers of population groups with diverse clinical problems that preclude comfortable wearing of complete dentures.[3-5]

Surgical placement of a number of implants into the anterior segments of the edentulous jaws has provided a method of support and retention of complete dentures where bone loss has depleted the denture-bearing areas. The number of implants used is dictated by bone quality and quantity and the success of the osseointegration process. Two or more implants used with a variety of available attachments or a retention bar system can assist denture retention and provide an improved quality of life for the patient (Fig 5-3).

Strategically placing five or six dental implants in one or both jaws has been very successful in providing totally edentulous patients with long-span fixed implant-supported prostheses, or overdentures retained by fixed

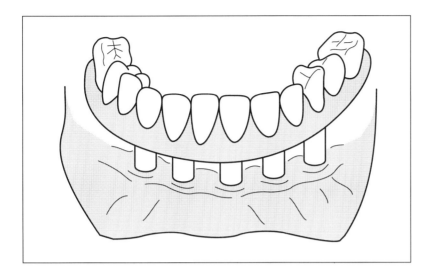

**Fig 5-2** Implant-supported fixed prosthesis placed in a totally edentulous mandible.

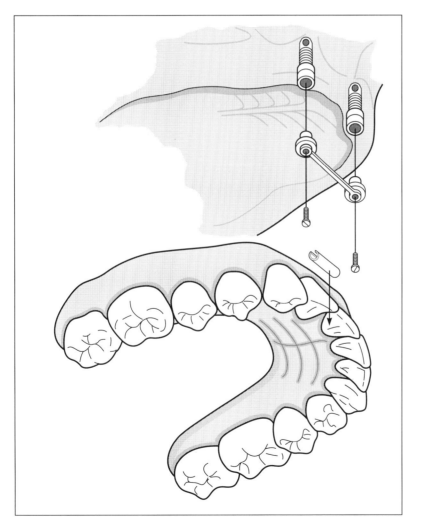

**Fig 5-3** Implant-supported overdenture. Retention is provided by the bar placed between two or more implants and the posterior residual alveolar ridge.

implant frameworks. Full-arch rehabilitations, using implants in both the maxilla and mandible with an appropriate selection of abutments and prosthesis designs, have contributed significantly to the improved comfort, function, and appearance of thousands of patients. The combination of implants and a fixed prosthesis in the mandibular arch with a maxillary denture has provided a major improvement in the dental health and overall well-being of many patients.

## Partially Edentulous Spaces Previously Occupied by More Than One Tooth

Dental implants have been used to restore partially edentulous spaces previously occupied by more than one natural tooth (Fig 5-4). The type, placement, and support of the prosthesis varies with the situation. For example, in the case of a missing central and lateral incisor in the maxillary anterior region, the prosthesis is most often attached only to the implants, and is a freestanding restoration. In other situations, the edentulous space may be longer and perhaps bounded at only one end by a natural tooth. These clinical situations often present numerous difficulties for conventional fixed or removable prosthodontic treatment, due to the root forms of the teeth adjacent to the edentulous space or to a variety of periodontal considerations.

The most frequently encountered partially edentulous situation is that of the patient with missing posterior dentitions in one or both quadrants. These situations are also the most difficult to treat because of the limitations caused by two anatomical structures, the maxillary sinus and the inferior alveolar nerve. A severely resorbed alveolar ridge or a large maxillary sinus may preclude the placement of implants in the lateral parts of the maxilla. For some patients, the canine area is sufficiently developed posteriorly and an implant can be placed in the first or second premolar area. The height of the alveolus below the floor of the sinus distal to the canine is usually less than 10 mm (Fig 5-5), which limits the number and type of implants that can be placed in that site. The most posterior part of the maxil-

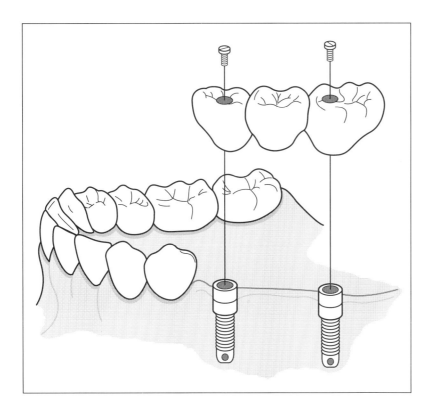

**Fig 5-4**   Implant-supported restoration in a partially edentulous mandible. This prosthesis is not usually attached to the adjoining natural tooth.

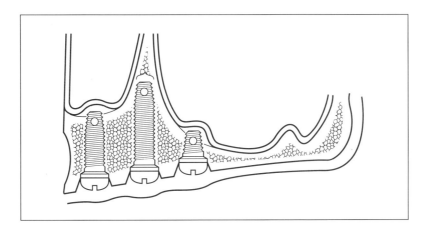

**Fig 5-5**   The amount of bone inferior to the maxillary sinus severely limits the potential for implant placement without additional surgical procedures. Note the difference in implant length from the anterior to the posterior maxilla.

lary arch, the tuberosity, usually has a sufficient quantity of bone, but this bone is too spongy to provide predictable osseointegration. However, the extremely dense mass of bone formed by the pterygoid process and the vertical part of the palatine bone distal to the tuberosity

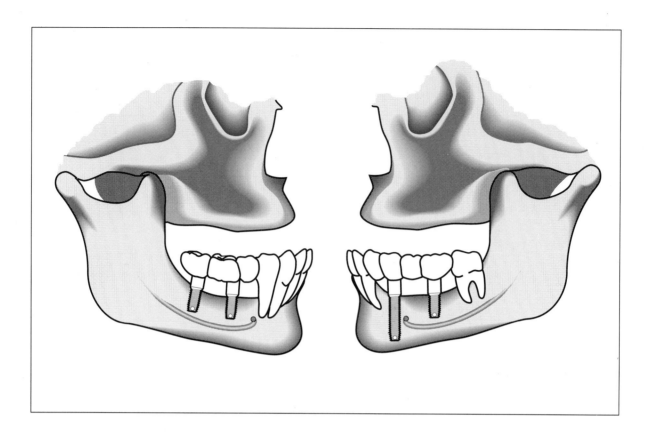

**Fig 5-6**   Placement of implants with respect to the mandibular canal. It is advisable to leave at least 1 mm of bone between the apex of the implant and the neurovascular bundle to prevent neural damage.

can sometimes provide better osseous support for implant placement. The volume of bone in the pterygomaxillary region has been found sufficient for implant placement in 80% of patient populations needing implants.[8]

In the mandible, the walls of the mandibular canal are usually clearly visible on radiographs, and it is not uncommon that both the volume and the density of bone above the mandibular canal are sufficient to provide anchorage for a 7-, 10- or even a 13-mm long implant (Fig 5-6). The difficulty in placing implants in these posterior areas is that of access, which consequently limits implant length. From the prosthodontic point of view, implants should not be placed beyond the area of the second molar if it is still present in the mouth. When the volume of bone above the canal is inadequate, there may still be enough bone lingual to the nerve for implant placement. However, the implant must engage the cortical bone inferiorly to achieve strong bicortical anchorage and almost certain osseointegration.

Two or more implants are normally used to restore the multiple-tooth edentulous area. The number of implants is an important consideration during treatment planning if the dentist is to provide a prosthesis that is freestanding and is not supported by natural teeth.

Joining natural teeth to the implant prosthesis may be an alternative; however, the clinical situation may exclude this treatment option. For example, if the prepared natural tooth and the implant do not draw, or cannot be seated together, elaborate mechanisms will be required to fix a prosthesis to the tooth and to the implant. These elaborate steps may even demand endodontic treatment to radically alter the direction of the coronal portion of the tooth. There have been questions as to the difference in mobility between natural teeth and osseointegrated implants, which may result in a loss of cementation between the implant prosthesis and the adjoining natural teeth. There are several prosthodontists who consider a crown on a natural tooth which is joined to an implant as part of the cantilever structure of the prosthesis, rather than part of its load-bearing support.

In the multiple-tooth implant prosthesis, a framework is fabricated to join the prosthesis to the implant abutments. The framework may be either a cast alloy or machined titanium. During the framework fabrication, various shapes of implant components are incorporated into the prosthesis framework; the type and configuration of these components are dependent upon customary prosthodontic concerns.

Patients in whom the loss of the bony ridge has created anatomical defects that adversely affect the potential for a successful result have benefited from bone grafting and/or guided tissue regeneration procedures used in conjunction with implants. These procedures can restore optimum ridge contours.

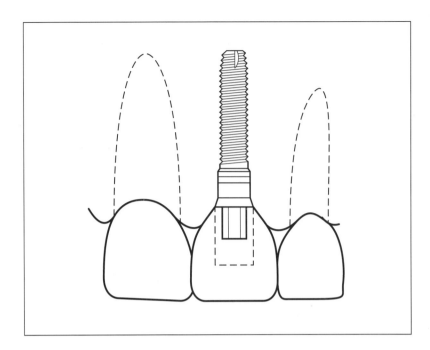

**Fig 5-7**    A single-tooth eden-tulous space restoration with an implant.

Dental implants have been used to restore the single-tooth edentulous space in situations where the natural tooth on either side is free of a dental restoration, or where the use of these natural teeth as abutments in conventional fixed prosthodontics is contraindicated (Fig 5-7). Using a single implant avoids the instrumentation of the natural teeth adjacent to the edentulous space. The use of dental implants is especially advantageous in situations in which the rotation and axial alignment of a potential abutment for a fixed partial denture would result in excess tissue reduction and might require endodontic therapy as part of the treatment plan.

Esthetic and biological demands of size and contour in the replacement restoration are important factors, and there are single-implant abutments designed to meet many different needs. Other important factors considered in the design of abutments for anterior single tooth replacements are the emergence angle and profile and conservation of space. Implant abutments are available that permit the creation of a crown that can be united with the implant abutment by a retention screw, or a crown design that can be cemented to the abutment.

Orthodontic tooth movement has always been limited to action-reaction reciprocal force mechanics because of the absence of a fixed anchorage point in the mouth. Extraoral headgear retraction of maxillary molars is currently the most effective way of obtaining anchorage for the orthodontic movement of teeth. Implants have been placed in the posterior mandible and used to protract the entire dentition in the maxilla and mandible.[9] Implants have been used effectively for retraction and correction of a Class III anterior crossbite malocclusion with missing molar teeth. Using implants for anchorage, orthodontic forces from 150 to 400 g were applied during the clinical course of treatment. The use of implants permits unidirectional tooth movement without reciprocal action. An implant may thus be used in place of molar teeth to act as anchors in the pushing and pulling of orthodontic treatment.

# Implants as Anchorage for Orthodontic Tooth Movement

Several treatment methods have been suggested to improve the denture-bearing area in patients with advanced atrophy of the edentulous mandible and maxilla. The most common methods are nonsurgical, surgical, or combinations of the two.

The nonsurgical approaches, even when conducted by the most skilled practitioners, have provided only limited improvement in the stability and retention of dentures for patients who lack bone support.

It is possible to improve the quantity, but not the quality, of bone in the mandible or maxilla by a surgical approach combining a vestibuloplasty and bone grafting.[10] Onlay autogenous or homogenous bone grafts have historically proven unpredictable from patient to patient. The long-term results for this method are rather discouraging; there is a 40% to 60% resorption of the bone graft during the first 2 years, and 60% to 100% loss by the end of 5 years.[11]

The technique of composite grafting, in which allogeneic material (hydroxyapatite) is added to the autogenous bone, initially showed promise. Unfortunately, graft

# Bone Grafting in Combination with Implants

displacement, irritability of the soft tissues by the allo-geneic material, and continued bone resorption in the placement site, limited the use of hydroxyapatite.[12]

Augmentation of the resorbed jaws using composite bone-grafting techniques has proven far more successful when combined with implants. These composite grafting procedures are performed in a hospital under a general anesthetic; and depending on the augmented site, involve either the onlay or inlay bone graft.

The necessary records for all potential graft patients include panoramic, lateral cephalometric, and occlusal radiographs, along with mounted diagnostic casts.[13,14] The patient's ability to tolerate the anesthetic and surgi-cal procedures must be determined. Psychological evalu-ations and testing are also recommended for these patients.

Sagittal and coronal compeuterized tomography (CT) scans have been suggested as a means of identifying the available basal bone for composite graft support. However, these scans are not considered essential in every case. A careful and detailed clinical examination and routine radiographic imaging may be all that is nec-essary for presurgical planning.

## Onlay Bone Grafting to the Mandible

The donor site most frequently used for the onlay graft is the iliac crest. The rib, tibia, and the mandibular symph-ysis are other suggested sites.

In the mandible, a mucoperiosteal incision which avoids the mental nerve is made along the length of the ridge crest, and the mandibular bone surface is prepared to receive the graft. A one-piece graft in the shape of a horseshoe is harvested from the iliac crest. After the bone is shaped for optimum contact with the residual ridge, it is rigidly fixed to the mandible using the appro-priate number of endosseous implants. Standard closure procedures are used for the surgical sites.

The optimum time required for remodeling of the graft and integration of the implants is still unknown, and the long-term follow-up studies evaluating this procedure are limited. However, resorption of the grafted bone appears to be less in the presence of implants, and an implant survival rate of 97.6% has been reported in grafted mandibles.[15,16] For these reasons, onlay bone grafting in combination with osseointegrated implants may be a valuable aid in the treatment of atrophic mandibles.

### Onlay Bone Grafting to the Maxilla

The amount of bone in the maxilla is limited by the midline nasal cavity and bilaterally by the maxillary sinuses; the bone quality is predominantly cancellous, rather than cortical. In situations of excessive bone resorption, several options have been suggested to increase the quantity of bone available in the maxilla for denture-base support.

Various types of composite grafts have been suggested as options with predictable outcomes. These include tibial cancellous bone chips packed around implants placed into residual maxillary bone, the preformed onlay composite tibial bone graft, and the onlay corticocancellous iliac bone graft.[1,17]

The 2-year implant survival rates for endosseous titanium implants used for graft anchorage with onlay grafts have been reported in the 80% to 90% range.[15,16,18,19]

Patients with advanced alveolar and basal bone resorption of the anterior and posterior maxilla may be candidates for the maxillary onlay composite graft. They usually have large antral and nasal cavities and minimal cortical bone thickness of the maxillary buttress, piriform aperture, and nasal floor. These patients must have adequate lip height to accommodate the onlay bone graft and eventually the prosthesis. If there is inadequate lip height, then the nasal-antral inlay composite graft technique should be considered.[20]

Assessing the health of the maxillary antrum of these patients is required because the bone graft-anchoring-endosseous implant will frequently violate the thin antral floor and lining membrane.

The intraoral incision is made high above the mucogingival junction of the maxillary edentulous ridge to allow for a watertight closure. Mucoperiosteal flaps are developed to expose the residual maxillary bone.

Once the graft is contoured and fitted properly to the residual maxillary defect, bone drilling procedures are carried out for placement of titanium implants through the graft and into the maxillary bone. Self-tapping implants are used in all maxillary composite graft patients.

### Inlay Bone Grafting to the Maxilla

Inlay bone grafting procedures should be considered in patients with both a short lip and alveolar bone loss. There is usually inadequate interarch space in these situations, and an inlay graft in the floor of the nose or antrum may be indicated, rather than the full-arch onlay composite graft.[21]

Adding bone to the superior surface of the maxilla or nasal floor provides an enclosed environment within the nasal cavity that is protected from the normal loading forces of a maxillary prosthesis.

The inlay bone graft is contoured to fit the floor of the nose or antrum and is fixed in position with endosseous implants, which extends through the residual ridge and into the inlay bone graft. When the floor of the nose is grafted, a Le Fort I osteotomy nasal exposure is performed and the rostrum and inferior septum are selectively removed. Cancellous particulate grafts, instead of block corticocancellous grafts, may also be used around the implants protruding above the nasal floor cortex. The antral grafts are placed through a lateral antral wall ostectomy or osteotomy with elevation of the Schneiderian membrane.

Multiple grafting regimens have been used to augment the sinus floor including maxillary osseous autografts and iliac onlay or inlay corticocancellous grafts, as well as other techniques.[22–24] The biological basis for osseous incorporation in the maxillary sinus area has not been well studied, although it is considered promising for maxillary downgrafting procedures.

The placement of implants into extraction sites immediately following the removal of periodontally involved teeth has been suggested as an alternative to waiting 6 to 12 months for bone healing to occur before placing the implants.[25] If enough bone exists below the apices of teeth that are to be extracted, then endosseous implants can be placed at the time of surgery. Although a higher failure rate for the immediate placement of implants has been observed, the practice appears to be reasonably safe and effective.

The advantages of immediate implant placement include decreased time from extraction to placement of the final prosthesis, fewer surgical procedures, and more favorable response by the patient to the overall treatment plan.

The disadvantages include the need for an interim prosthesis during the healing phase and a potentially greater risk of infection. There are inherently more bacteria present in a mouth with periodontally involved teeth than in a completely edentulous mouth, and contamination of the surgical site during immediate implant placement is a distinct possibility.[26] More clinical studies are needed to validate the benefits of immediate implants, and to determine the mechanisms of failure.

# Immediate Implant Placement

A factor of extreme importance in the clinical application of implants in the anterior region of the mouth is inadequate bone in the implant site adjacent to natural teeth. To generate bone adjacent to the implant, guided tissue regeneration has been suggested as an adjunct to implant treatment. This procedure is based on the regeneration of periodontal structures using progenitor cells, which have the potential to form cementum, the periodontal ligament, and alveolar bone, to repopulate a bony defect. Cells that are not capable of rebuilding periodontal tissues are excluded from contaminating the healing wound. Physical barriers in the form of membranes are used to prevent epithelial cells and cells originating from the connective tissue from migrating into

# Guided Tissue Regeneration

the wound. According to this principle, a selective osteogenesis within a defined defect can be accomplished.

The guidance of cell ingrowth originating from bone is accomplished by isolating the defect from the adjacent epithelial tissues with a membrane having a pore size that will not allow the penetration of cells. Additionally, a space is created into which progenitor cells capable of inducing bone formation can migrate, proliferate, and differentiate into osteoblasts and osteocytes. When the space between the membrane and the implant is stabilized with new bone growth, the membrane is removed. Using this membrane technique, complete bone regeneration of bone defects around implants has been achieved.[27-29] Further research to expand the potential of guided tissue regeneration is needed.

# References

1. Brånemark P-I. Introduction to osseointegration. In: Brånemark P-I, Zarb GA, Albrektsson T (eds). Tissue-Integrated Prostheses: Osseointegration in Clinical Dentistry. Chicago: Quintessence, 1985:11–77.

2. Schnitman PA, Shulman LB. Recommendations on the consensus development conference on dental implants. J Am Dent Assoc 1979; 98:373.

3. Adell R, Eriksson B, Lekholm U, Brånemark P-I, Jemt T. A long-term follow-up study of osseointegrated implants in the treatment of totally edentulous jaws. Int J Oral Maxillofac Implants 1990;5:347–359.

4. Adell R, Lekholm U, Rockler BR, Brånemark P-I. A 15-year study of osseointegrated implants in the treatment of the edentulous jaw. Int J Oral Surg 1981;10:387–416.

5. Albrektsson T, Bergman B, Folmer T, Henry PJ, Higuchi K, Klineberg I et al. A multicenter report of osseointegrated oral implants. J Prosthet Dent 1988;60:75–84.

6. Meskin LH, Brown LJ, Brunell JA, Warren GB. Patterns of tooth loss and accumulated prosthetic treatment potential in U.S. employed adults and seniors 1985–86. Gerodontics 1988; 4:126–135.

7. Douglass CW. Clinical practice: Deliver of services. Review of the literature. J Prosthet Dent 1990;64:274–283.

8.  Tulasne J-F. Implant treatment of missing posterior dentition. In: Laney WR, Tolman DE (eds). Tissue Integration in Oral, Orthopedic, and Maxillofacial Reconstruction. Chicago: Quintessence, 1992:103–105.

9.  Higuchi K, Slack JM. The use of titanium fixtures for intraoral anchorage to facilitate orthodontic tooth movement. In: Laney WR, Tolman DE (eds). Tissue Integration in Oral, Orthopedic, and Maxillofacial Reconstruction. Chicago: Quintessence, 1992:303–307.

10. Hillerup S, Eriksen E, Solow B. Reduction of mandibular residual ridge after vestibuloplasty. A two-year follow-up study comparing the Edian flap, mucosal and skin graft operations. Int J Oral Maxillofac Surg 1989;18:271–276.

11. Davis DM. The role of implants in the treatment of edentulous patients. Int J Prosthodont 1990;3:42–50.

12. Desjardins RP. Hydroxylapatite for alveolar ridge augmentation: Indications and problems. J Prosthet Dent 1985;54:374–388.

13. Eckerdal O, Kvint S. Presurgical planning for osseointegrated implants in the maxilla. J Oral Maxillofac Surg 1986;15:722–726.

14. Laney WR. Selecting edentulous patients for tissue-integrated prostheses. Int J Oral Maxillofac Implants 1986;1:129–138.

15. Albrektsson T, Dahl E, Enbom L, Engevall S, Engquist B, Ericsson AR et al. Osseointegrated oral implants. A Swedish multicenter study of 8139 consecutively inserted Nobelpharma implants. J Periodontol 1988;59:287–296.

16. Albrektsson T. A multicenter report on osseointegrated oral implants. J Prosthet Dent 1988;60:75–84.

17. Brånemark P-I, Lekholm U. Tissue-integrated prostheses in oral and maxillofacial reconstruction. In: Levin N (ed). Current Treatment in Dental Practice. Philadelphia: Saunders, 1986:359, 361–362.

18. Kahnberg KE, Nystrom E, Bartholdsson L. Combined use of bone grafts and Brånemark fixtures in the treatment of severely resorbed maxillae. Int J Oral Maxillofac Implants 1989; 4:297–304.

19. Adell R, Lekholm U, Grondahl K, Brånemark P-I, Lindstrom J, Jacobsson M. Reconstruction of severely resorbed edentulous maxillae using osseointegrated fixtures in immediate autogenous bone grafts. Int J Oral Maxillofac Implants 1990;5:233–245.

20. Jensen J, Krantz Simonsen E, Sindet-Pedersen S. Reconstruction of the severely resorbed maxilla with bone grafting and osseointegrated implants. A preliminary report. J Oral Maxillofac Surg 1990;48:27–32.

21. Tolman DE, Desjardins RP, Keller EE. Surgical-prosthodontic reconstruction of oronasal defects utilizing the tissue-integrated prosthesis. Int J Oral Maxillofac Implants 1988;3:31–40.

22. Kent J, Block M. Simultaneous maxillary sinus floor bone grafting and placement of hydroxylapatite-coated implants. J Oral Maxillofac Surg 1989;47:238–242.

23. Wood RM, Moore DL. Grafting of the maxillary sinus with intraorally harvested autogenous bone prior to implant placement. Int J Oral Maxillofac Implants 1988;3:211–214.

24. Jensen OT, Greer R. Immediate placement of osseointegrating implants into the maxillary sinus augmented with mineralized cancellous allograft and Gore-Tex: Second-stage surgical and histological findings. In: Laney WR, Tolman DE (eds). Tissue Integration in Oral, Orthopedic, and Maxillofacial Reconstruction. Chicago: Quintessence, 1992:321–333.

25. Krump JL, Barnett BG. The immediate implant: A treatment alternative. Int J Oral Maxillofac Implants 1991;6:19–23.

26. Dzink JL, Tanner ACR, Haffajee AD, Socransky SS. Gram negative species associated with active destructive periodontal lesions. J Clin Periodontol 1985;12:648–659.

27. Wachtel HC, Langford A. Guided bone regeneration next to osseointegrated implants in humans. Int J Oral Maxillofac Implants 1991;6:127–135.

28. Dahlin C, Sennerby L, Lekholm U, Linde A, Nyman S. Generation of new bone around titanium implants using a membrane technique: An experimental study in rabbits. Int J Oral Maxillofac Implants 1989;4:19–25.

29. Dahlin C, Gottlow J, Linde A, Nyman S. Healing of bone defects by guided tissue regeneration. Plast Reconstr Surg 1988; 81(5):672–676.

# 6

# Extraoral Implant Applications

*Michael R. Arcuri*
*Michael E. Razzoog*

## Prosthetic Treatment of Craniofacial Defects

The extraoral implant differs in design from those used intraorally. Due to the thinner bone found around the ear, orbit, and midface, extraoral implants are considerably shorter than intraoral implants, typically 3, 4, or 5 mm in length, with a circumferential flange (Fig 6-1). The flange adds to the surface area of the implant, providing better bone contact.

There are many ways in which osseointegrated implants can be used to correct defects in the head and neck (Fig 6-2). In 1979, at the University of Gothenburg in Sweden, the first bone-anchored ear prosthesis was placed.[1] Implants have been used in bone-conduction hearing aids, which conduct sound to the auditory nerves directly through the cranium. This procedure was first done at the University of Gothenburg in 1977. Incorporation of microcircuitry into implants to reduce the size and improve the quality of these hearing aids is yet to be explored.

Eye prostheses may also be affixed with implants. Implant anchorage in the zygoma, frontal bones, and maxilla presents many opportunities for facial reconstruction. Implants have been used in treating bone fractures, and it has been suggested that implants may be used to expand areas of the face or skull. Implants may be used in the future to replace diseased temporomandibular joints.

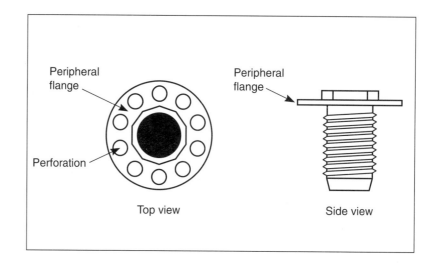

**Fig 6-1** A screw-type implant for extraoral applications. Note the peripheral flange, which aids retention in thinner bone.

Although the advantages of craniofacial implant applications have been demonstrated, a number of applications do not currently have approval from the Food and Drug Administration.

With the use of extraoral implants, patients claim that their prostheses remain more secure, thus giving them more confidence in public settings. Without the use of adhesives, the placement and removal of prostheses is greatly simplified, and the lifespan of prostheses is increased.

## Prosthetic Joint Replacements

Trauma, loss of limb, birth defects, and osteoarthrosis have increased the need for prosthetic joint replacements followed by reconstruction and rehabilitation. Implants have been used in a select number of patients needing artificial joints. An artificial joint must provide fixation for an endoprosthesis. The joint mechanism must be uncomplicated, and the replacement of the joint mechanism must be simple should the mechanism fail or should an improved version become available. The results using implants have been most promising, and the need for more research and further clinical trials is clear.

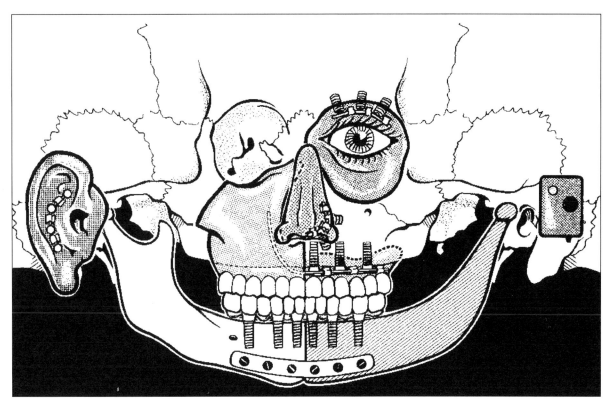

**Fig 6.2**  Summary of the possible uses for osseointegrated implants in the oral and maxillofacial region. (Reprinted by permission of Dr P.-I. Brånemark.)

Trauma or surgery for tumor removal may result in defects of the maxilla or mandible that affect function and esthetics. When radiotherapy is used for cancer treatment, the quality of the irradiated bone is decreased. While these patients with defects of the maxilla or mandible would benefit from implant treatment, they are also most at risk for implant failure due to radiotherapy.

Radiotherapy causes a decrease in the quality and quantity of saliva, a reduction in the blood supply to the irradiated tissues, and a decrease in the ability for bone to remodel and repair itself. The resulting poor healing capacities of irradiated tissues can impede osseointegration. Bacterial invasion into the bony defect left after removal of the fixture can progress to osteoradionecrosis.

# Discontinuity Defects and Healing-Impaired Patients

This condition, although rarely life-threatening, sometimes requires surgical resection of the involved tissues.

A hyperbaric oxygen (HBO) protocol has been developed to reduce these complications.[2] The protocol requires 20 preoperative and 10 postoperative sessions, in which the patient breathes 100% oxygen for 90 minutes at 2.4 atmospheres. The HBO therapy causes an increase in the microvascular blood supply to the irradiated tissues. The placement of implants into irradiated tissues in conjunction with HBO therapy has produced some promising results. However, the placement of implants into irradiated bone should not be considered a routine procedure at this time.

# References

1.  Tjellström A, Jacobsson M. The Bone-Anchored Maxillofacial Prosthesis. In: Albrektsson T, Zarb GA (eds). The Brånemark Osseointegrated Implant. Chicago: Quintessence, 1989:235–244.

2.  Marx RE, Ames JR. The use of hyperbaric oxygen therapy in bony reconstruction of the irradiated and tissue deficient patient. J Oral Maxillofacial Surgery 1982;40:412–420.

# Diagnostics and Treatment Planning

*Michael R. Arcuri*
*Brien R. Lang*

## Patient Selection

To determine if a patient is a candidate for implant therapy, a thorough review of the medical and dental history is important. Certain medical conditions may preclude the patient from undergoing implant treatment; these are discussed in the next section. The dental history may give some insight to the patient's previous prosthetic experiences, dental knowledge, and expectations.

The patient who, when seeking evaluation for implant therapy, presents the clinician with a bag of recently fabricated prostheses, or who wears mismatched sets of dentures, may have unrealistic expectations. Patients who claim they have "special needs" and express great doubt that anyone can successfully treat them may also be poor candidates for implants. These types of patients may also turn out to be successful implant patients, but they may require additional diagnostic procedures, such as trial dentures, and education prior to implant therapy.

In evaluating a partially edentulous patient for implants, several questions should be discussed:

1. Would the missing tooth structure be better replaced by a fixed partial denture?
2. Does an acceptable occlusal plane exist or could one be developed in conjunction with implant treatment?
3. Does adequate interarch space exist for the implant restoration?
4. Does adequate intertooth distance exist for placement of an implant and restoration?

Longstanding short edentulous spaces might be better suited for restoration with a fixed partial denture rather than with implants. This type of area often has bony topography containing buccal concavities, which may make successful placement of an implant difficult because of limited available bone (Fig 7-1).

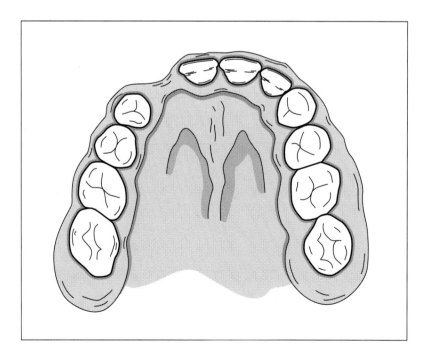

**Fig 7-1**   A long-term extraction site displays severe resorption of the alveolar ridge, making implant placement problematic.

Irregular cusp heights in the posterior dentition may result in occlusal prematurities and excursive interferences during lateral jaw movements that could result in excessive stresses being transmitted to the implants. These stresses may decrease the long-term success of the implant.

If inadequate space exists for implant placement, damage to adjacent tooth-root structures may occur. Close coronal proximity to adjacent teeth may force the development of less-than-optimal embrasure and occlusal contours in the restoration. Inadequate inter-arch space may make fabrication of the restoration difficult, producing less-than-optimal esthetic and functional results.

Good oral hygiene is necessary for long-term implant success, but completely or partially edentulous patients with extremely poor oral hygiene should not be excluded from implant treatment. After educating such patients about the significance of good oral hygiene, however, it is advisable that a trial period of several months be undertaken. If the patient achieves and maintains adequate hygiene levels during this time, the patient could then be considered for implant treatment.

A preliminary radiographic study is important during the initial patient evaluation. It may give indications of the quantity and quality of bone available for implant placement. These initial radiographs may include but are not limited to panoramic, occlusal, and periapical radiographs. Additional radiographic analysis may include the use of computerized tomography (CT) scans.

Prior to acceptance of a patient for treatment, a diagnostic waxup with articulated casts should be performed. This will provide information for the clinician and technician on the feasibility of developing a successful restoration. The diagnostic casts may also be shown to the patient to demonstrate the type of restoration planned (fixed or removable) and areas of possible complications.

Pretreatment evaluations vary from patient to patient. Some of the more common steps in this process are the following:

1. Medical and dental histories
2. Complete oral and dental examinations
3. Radiographic examinations
4. Psychological evaluation
5. Mounted diagnostic casts
6. Diagnostic waxup
7. Template for surgical procedure
8. Signed informed consent

The final step prior to accepting a patient for treatment is to ensure that the patient understands the procedures, timing of treatment, projected treatment outcomes, and cost. It is important that the patient understands the need for routine follow-up visits and possible periodic maintenance of the prosthesis.

# Indications and Contraindications

As long-term studies on implant therapy have progressed, it has become apparent that the placement of an endosseous implant not only provides a source of retention and stability for a prosthesis, but generates some stimulation to the surrounding bone. This stimulation appears to inhibit the alveolar resorption that follows tooth extraction, which has been described as both chronic and irreversible, and whose long-term effects produce numerous morphological changes that adversely affect denture-bearing areas and facial esthetics. By decreasing resorption, an implant provides a system for bone maintenance, enhancing the therapeutic value of implant treatment.

Indications for implant therapy in an edentulous alveolus could include any patient who meets the following requirements:

1. Has adequate quality and quantity of bone available for implant placement.
2. Is healthy enough to undergo the surgical procedure.
3. Is able to maintain optimal levels of oral hygiene.
4. Is psychologically stable and understands implant therapy, its limitations, and the patient's responsibilities.

Opinions on the minimal quantity of bone required for implant placement vary; however, the following are general considerations:

1. 6 mm buccal-lingual width
2. 8 mm interradicular bone width
3. 10 mm alveolar bone above the inferior alveolar canal or below the maxillary sinus

Because the indications for implant therapy are extremely broad, an analysis of contraindications may be more useful for determining if this treatment is suitable for a patient. Some of these contraindications are also discussed in the following section on patient examination. With few exceptions, contraindications are relative parameters and not absolute guidelines.

*Anatomical contraindications* are dictated by the availability of alveolar bone in which to place the implants. Inadequate height and/or width of the residual alveolus may make placement of the implants entirely within bone impossible. This may result in the ingrowth of fibrous connective tissue between the implant and bone, inhibiting osseointegration. Minimal cortical plate thickness and low-density trabecular bone may make initial stabilization of the implant difficult and long-term osseointegration questionable.

*Medical contraindications* primarily concern the ability of the patient's tissues to heal. Implants should not be placed while a patient is undergoing treatments that cause a systemic impairment of healing, such as chemotherapy for the treatment of cancer and antimetabolic therapy (eg, methotrexate) for the treatment of arthritis. Patients who suffer from uncontrolled diabetes should also forego implant treatment until the disease is properly managed, as should patients with seriously impaired cardiovascular function. Active addictions to drugs, including alcohol, should also be considered medical contraindications to treatment with implants.

Patients with a history of radiation therapy to the maxillomandibular region should not be considered for implant treatment under routine protocols. Implants may be successfully placed in irradiated bone, but the procedures for placement and restoration of the implants are still in the investigative phase of development.

*Psychiatric contraindications* are often the most difficult ones to identify. These conditions may be undiagnosed or unreported by the patient. Blomberg[1] has identified the following as psychiatric contraindications to treatment:

1. Psychotic syndromes, such as schizophrenia or paranoia

2. Severe character disorders and neurotic syndromes, such as hysteroid and borderline personality disorders

3. Dysmorphophobia (an irrational fear of deformity), and patients with extreme and unrealistic expectations and demands regarding the cosmetic results of the operation, rather than the effects of retention problems

4. Syndromes of cerebral lesions and presenile dementia

5. Alcohol or drug abuse, if not diagnosed with great certainty as secondary to the oral problem

In general, the absence of one or more teeth may be an indication for implant therapy, providing the patient understands the treatment, is able to maintain the prosthesis hygienically, and has no factors that would impair the development of osseointegration.

# Presentation of the Treatment Plan to the Patient

If there are no contraindications to implants, the treatment plan, including the numbers and kinds of prosthetic improvements planned and the overall cost, should be presented in detail to the patient. The patient's esthetic and functional desires must be discussed and evaluated to determine if he or she has unrealistic expectations. A careful evaluation of the patient's willingness and ability to provide the necessary home care before, during, and after active treatment is also necessary. Some decisions, such as whether the implant prosthesis will be fixed or removable, or whether a single implant crown will be screwed or cemented in place, may not be possible at this time and may need to be deferred until the actual therapy is in progress. The patient should be thoroughly informed about these issues, all of which must be resolved before surgery.

# An Outline for Implant Therapy

**1. The Patient Examination**
   The General Health
   The Dental Health
   Radiographic Evaluations
   Photographic Record

**2. The Diagnostic Mounting**

**3. Presentation of the Treatment Plan to the Patient**

**4. Stage I Surgery: Implant Placement**
   Healing Period
      • 3-month minimum for the mandible
      • 6-month minimum for the maxilla
   Prosthodontic Procedures

**5. Stage II Surgery: Abutment Placement**
   Healing Period
      • 2 to 3 weeks before start of definitive prosthodontic care
   Prosthodontic Procedures

**6. Definitive Prosthodontic Treatment**

**7. Periodic Recall Appointments and Maintenance Program**

The patient's past medical and dental history, a hard and soft tissue examination, radiographic evaluations of the jaw under consideration for implants provide valuable patient data. A diagnostic cast mounted on a semiadjustable articulator and intra-and extraoral photographs are essential to developing the treatment plan and to sequencing the treatment. The patient examination should address factors of general and oral health, as well as the morphological features of the proposed edentulous site for implant placement.

# Patient Examination

## General Health

The clinician should screen for any disease process that would compromise complete healing. Controlled diabetes, osteoporosis, and various cardiovascular diseases might be causes for concern, but these diseases have not been reported as contraindicating implant treatment,[2] and when present, usually require only that conventional precautions be followed throughout surgical intervention to assure success. Neither age nor prolonged steroid use are considered factors that would eliminate a patient from implant therapy.

Patients with impaired psychological function and personality patterns of avoidance behavior should be thoroughly reviewed by appropriate medical colleagues before they are accepted as implant candidates. Psychiatric contraindications, such as those listed above, should cause the dentist to question implant therapy as the treatment of choice for these patients. Chemical dependencies, for example, may prevent patients' compliance and oral hygiene motivation for a complex reconstruction including dental implants.

Patients in reasonably good general health and who appear psychologically stable are good candidates for implants. Above all else, patients must demonstrate that they are motivated to pursue treatment and that they will cooperate with recommendations made by clinicians.

## Dental Health

The condition of the mucous membranes, the health of the jaws, and the status of any remaining teeth are the primary local health factors to be considered. Healthy oral mucosa is a required criterion in implant placement, and any soft or hard tissue pathosis must be dealt with before implant therapy can be considered. Herpetic stomatitis, candidiasis, denture-induced stomatitis, and hyperplastic tissues are examples of inflammatory conditions that negatively influence treatment success. Tooth impactions, bone cysts, root fragments, and residual bone infections contraindicate implant therapy, and the presence of a benign bone tumor in the jaw would also eliminate a patient from implant treatment.

Every edentulous space has the potential of being restored with the aid of dental implants; however, all reasonable types of prosthetic reconstructive procedures must be considered during the examination. Implants are only one option among the many types of prosthodontic services available. The prosthetic choices are influenced by the adjacent teeth with respect to their periodontal health and the presence or absence of existing restorations. The pulpal health, esthetic requirements, and shape and contours of the residual ridge in the edentulous space can also affect the decision. The alignment and orientation of the adjacent teeth can also be an influence.

The oral examination should include measurements of any edentulous spaces.[3] Spaces 7 mm or more wide between neighboring teeth are considered acceptable for single implant placement; a space of 6 mm is regarded as the minimum treatable space. A minimum vertical interarch distance of 5 mm is needed for the implant prosthetic components. The vertical difference between the gingival margin of the neighboring teeth and the top of the ridge crest in the edentulous space is another measurement that should be recorded. In situations with an excessively resorbed ridge, a greater vertical difference will result in the need for a very long clinical crown, which may compromise the eventual esthetic results.

## Radiographic Evaluations

A panoramic radiograph (orthopanograph) is the first step in evaluating bone quantity and quality in the potential implant site; however, definitive determination of the quantity and quality of bone should not be made from this alone. The nature of the cortical and cancellous (spongy) portion of the bone sites cannot be accurately detected from the orthopanograph, and there are also significant distortions of spatial relationships in this type of radiograph.

A lateral jaw cephalogram gives a better indication of the thickness of cortical bone and the amount and nature of cancellous bone in the midline, with less spatial distortion than in the orthopanograph. The cephalogram provides valuable information about the contour of the anterior alveolar ridge, the prominence of the genial tubercle, the location of the mandibular canal and mental foramina, and the spatial relationship of the patient's jaws.

The periapical radiographic survey provides valuable information about the health, root forms and contours, and bone support of the remaining teeth. An occlusal radiograph will give some information about the width of the bone in the implant placement site.

Radiographic information is extremely important in decisions regarding implant treatment and the overall treatment plan for the patient. With those patients in whom it is difficult to adequately judge the shape of the residual bone morphology, CT scans may also be helpful.

Lekholm and Zarb have attempted to classify the bone quantity and quality in the edentulous mandible and maxilla as a guide for selection of patients for osseointegrated implants.[4] The bone shape or quantity assessments are presented in Figure 7-2 and are rated from A through E. The assessment of bone quality is presented in Figure 7-3; a rating from 1 through 4 describes the amount of compact and cancellous bone present in the edentulous jaw.

Certain combinations of bone quantity and quality provide a potentially better prognosis for implant survival than others. For example, a patient with a B or

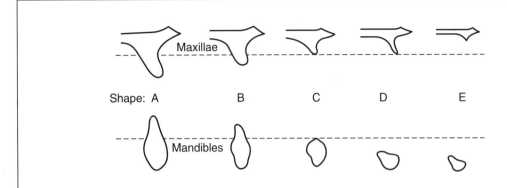

Shape: A    B    C    D    E

**A.** Most of the alveolar ridge is present.

**B.** Moderate alveolar ridge resorption has occurred.

**C.** Advanced alveolar ridge resorption has occurred and only basal bone remains.

**D.** Some resorption of the basal bone has taken place.

**E.** Extreme resorption of the basal bone has taken place.

**Fig 7-2**   Bone quantity.

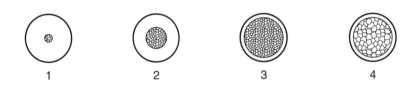

1    2    3    4

**1.** Almost the entire jaw is comprised of homogenous compact bone.

**2.** A thick layer of compact bone surrounds a core of dense trabecular bone.

**3.** A thin layer of cortical bone surrounds a core of dense trabecular bone of favorable strength.

**4.** A thin layer of cortical bone surrounds a core of low density trabecular bone.

**Fig 7-3**   Bone quality.

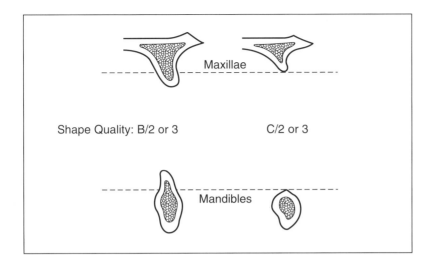

**Fig 7-4a**   Optimum shapes and qualities of bone for implant placement in maxillary and mandibular bone.

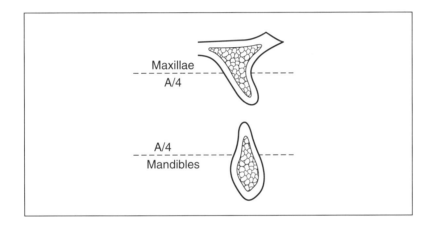

**Fig 7-4b**   Low density or poor quality bone. Osseointegration in this type of bone is questionable, especially in the maxilla.

C bone quantity and a 2 or 3 bone quality would have a more favorable prognosis than a patient with an A bone quantity and a 4 bone quality (Figs 7-4a and b). In the latter situation, the residual ridge consists of a thin layer of cortical bone surrounding trabecular bone of unfavorable strength and low density, which leads to instability during both the drilling and the implant placement procedures.

Even though a great deal of information can be gained from the radiographic evaluations, the final decision on implant placement will rest with the surgeon at the time of surgery, when the true quantity and quality of the bone can be determined.

**Photographs**

Intraoral and extraoral photographs have proven invaluable as a record of pretreatment conditions. They are also important as a visual record during the treatment planning stages of implant therapy.

## The Implant Team: The Key to Success

It is important that all members of the clinical team cooperate from the beginning of treatment planning. General dentists, oral surgeons, periodontists, and prosthodontists all contribute to implant success, and need to communicate with each other before, during, and after active therapy. This approach reflects the basic philosophical tenet established by Brånemark that regardless of the implant system used, the concept of a team approach to patient care is of paramount importance. The combined team efforts of surgical and restorative personnel from the beginning of therapy are essential ingredients for success. Sharing as much information as possible among all treatment personnel will increase the chances for implant success. The specific roles of each member of the implant team will be discussed in greater detail as the specific steps in implant therapy are explained.

Osseointegration is a significant addition to the options available to patients and practitioners for solving problems of partial and total edentulism. Implants provide another treatment option for the patient with a periodontally compromised dentition. With the flexibility to replace natural teeth that are failing periodontally by a succession of osseointegrated implants, periodontists realize that total edentulism is no longer the ultimate limiting factor in periodontal treatment. Implants provide a new dimension in prosthodontic treatment options, from single-tooth applications to complex periodontal restorative situations to management of the totally edentulous patient.

The decision to conserve the residual structures through the earlier loss of hopeless teeth and to replace these teeth with freestanding implant-supported restorations is difficult. An alternative is to continue the patient in a "holding pattern" of care that will eventually result in the loss of teeth and an even greater loss of supporting structures. To the conservative-minded general dentist, providing patients with implants as treatment solutions may be most difficult. However, general dentists must be prepared to fulfill the requirements for proper informed consent. Dentists must be ready to embrace the team concept and to provide implant treatment, or be willing to refer the patient to others who are trained in and use these techniques.

No dental professional can function in isolation. Whether one is an oral surgeon, periodontist, prosthodontist, or general dentist, one must function as members of a patient-care team, cooperating in diagnosis, treatment planning, surgical procedures, restorations, and maintenance of implants and general oral health. Dentists and their patients have previously suffered from the limitations and uncertainties of an unknown prognosis with implants; however, the concept and principles of osseointegration and the team approach have reversed this situation. Treatment is now predictable, with long-term success its continuing outcome.

# References

1. Blomberg S. Psychological response. In: Brånemark P-I, Zarb GA, Albrektsson T (eds). Tissue-Integrated Prostheses: Osseointegration in Clinical Dentistry. Chicago: Quintessence, 1985:165–164.

2. Laney WR, Tolman DE. The Mayo Clinic experience with tissue-integrated prostheses. In: Albrektsson T, Zarb GA (eds). The Brånemark Osseointegrated Implant. Chicago: Quintessence, 1989:165–195.

3. Lekholm U, Jemt T. Principles for single tooth replacement. In: Albrektsson T, Zarb GA (eds). The Brånemark Osseointegrated Implant. Chicago: Quintessence, 1989:117–126.

4. Lekholm U, Zarb GA. Patient selection and preparation. In: Brånemark P-I, Zarb GA, Albrektsson T (eds). Tissue-Integrated Prostheses: Osseointegration in Clinical Dentistry. Chicago: Quintessence, 1985:199–209.

# 8

# The Surgical Stages of Osseointegration

*Philip Worthington*

The surgical stages of osseointegration, in which implants are introduced into the jaw, will now be described in detail. These standardized surgical procedures are directly related to the basic research performed by P.-I. Brånemark and his coworkers in Sweden, and they derive from an understanding of wound healing in general and bone biology in particular.

For the most commonly used endosseous implant systems, the surgery is performed in two stages separated in time by a few months.[1]

The first surgical stage may be performed under local or general anesthesia and involves the preparation of the implant sites in the jaw bone and the introduction of the implants into the bone in a way that inflicts minimal trauma on the tissues. The soft tissues are then closed and the implants are thus excluded from the mouth. During the healing period that follows implant placement, the implants should be protected from transmitted pressure, such as that which might come from an overlying denture. This time allows the bone to heal and osseointegration to occur; the healing bone grows up to and adheres to the layer of titanium oxides or ceramic coating, such as hydroxyapatite, on the surface of the implant. In the mandible, this period will be a minimum of 3 months long. In the maxilla, it will be a minimum of

6 months long, because of the looser texture and slower healing of the maxillary bone.

In the second stage of surgery, the buried implant is exposed and a cylindrical titanium abutment, which protrudes into the mouth, is connected to it. This abutment will serve as the attachment for the prosthesis, which is fabricated by the restorative dentist or prosthodontist.

# Stage I Surgery: Placement of the Implants

The bone of the jaw is exposed by the reflection of a flap of mucoperiosteum and a potential implant site is identified and marked with a small round bur (Figs 8-1a and b). The next step is to drill a narrow cylindrical hole in the bone using a twist drill (Fig 8-1c). Care must be taken to control the angulation of the drill, bearing in mind the future prosthodontic needs. This narrow cylindrical hole is then widened, first using a pilot drill that has a blunt tip and a wider cutting blade behind that, then using a wide twist drill to widen the hole to the required depth (Fig 8-1d). A countersink is then used to shape the upper part of the bone to receive the flared neck of the implant (Fig 8-1e). All these steps are performed using drill speeds below 2,000 revolutions per minute and using profuse saline irrigation for cooling.

After measuring the depth of the implant site with a special measuring gauge, the preparation is completed by using a titanium tap to cut a thread on the walls of the cylindrical hole (Fig 8-1f). A special drill, rotating at no more than 15 revolutions per minute, is used. This step is also performed with cooling irrigation.

When the implant site is thus prepared, an implant can be threaded into it and gently screwed into place (Fig 8-1g). The aim is to place a series of implants in the edentulous jaw with near parallelism; absolute parallelism is not essential. For a close approximation of parallelism, the surgeon uses metal direction indicators temporarily placed in the initial drill holes. In this way, the operator can judge the angulation of the next implant to be placed in sequence.

When all the implants are in the bone, the final step is to put a cover screw in the top of each implant (Fig 8-1h)

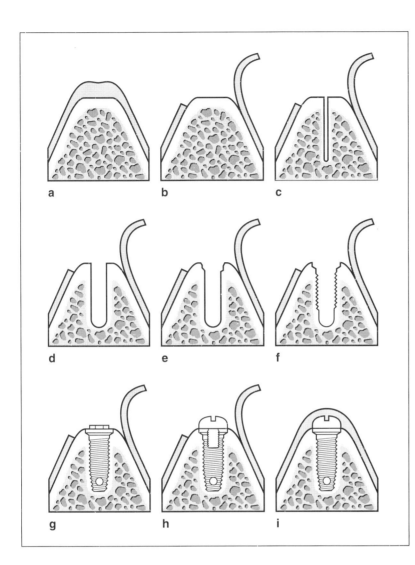

**Fig 8-1**  Stage I surgery for 2-stage implant endosseous implant systems. The preoperative alveolar ridge appears in cross-section *(a)*. The mucoperiosteal flap is raised *(b)* and an initial hole is drilled into the bone *(c)*. This hole is then widened *(d)* and usually modified with a countersinking drill *(e)*. This hole is then threaded with a tap *(f)*. The implant is gently screwed into place *(g)* and a cover screw added to occlude the central space *(h)*. The mucosal flap can then be replaced to exclude the implant from the oral cavity during the healing period *(i)*.

so as to occlude its internal thread and to prevent connective tissue and bone form growing over and obscuring the occlusal end of the implant.

The mucoperiosteal tissue flap is then replaced and sutured in position (Fig 8-1i). The patient should not wear a denture over the operated site for about 2 weeks. At the end of that time, the denture may be modified by the restorative dentist; the flanges can be reduced, the fitting surface can be relieved at the implant sites, and the whole fitting surface can be coated with a soft lining material. The patient may then wear the modified denture during the few months of the bone-healing period.

# Stage II Surgery: The Abutment Connection

First, the buried implants are located by palpation and, if necessary, by probing. Under local anesthesia, they are then exposed by means of a mucoperiosteal incision and, if necessary, by using a circular punch to remove overlying mucoperiosteum. This exposure allows the surgeon to remove the cover screws and to make sure that the upper end of each implant is clean and free from overlying wisps of connective tissue and bone. The depth of the mucoperiosteum is measured, and an abutment cylinder of suitable length is chosen and connected to the implant using an abutment screw and a small screwdriver (Fig 8-2a). At this stage the abutment cylinder protrudes into the mouth and the surrounding gingiva may be replaced and sutured in position. When all the abutment cylinders have been placed, healing caps are attached to their occlusal ends to allow a temporary periodontal pack to be placed and retained. This protects the gingiva and holds the mucoperiosteal flap against the bone. Accurate seating of the abutment cylinders is checked both visually in the mouth and by radiographs. This is the first time since implant placement that a radiograph is permitted.

After a week or two, the pack and the sutures are removed and the patient is ready to begin the restorative phase of treatment, which involves mounting of the prosthetic components (Figs 8-2b and c).

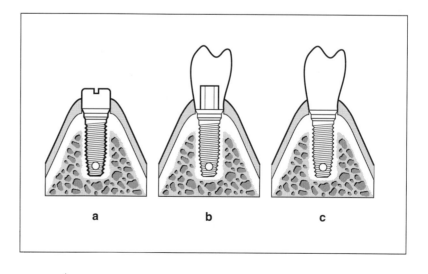

**Fig 8-2**   Stage 2 surgery for 2-stage endosseous implant systems. The cover screws are located, removed, and replaced by an abutment cylinder that penetrates the mucosa into the mouth *(a)*. The prosthetic component is then mounted on the abutment *(b),* and the final restoration is attached with a screw or cement *(c)*.

a          b          c

# Keys to Implant Surgery Success

1. **Minimize the risk of infection by:**
   a. Careful preparation and draping of the patient
   b. Sterile technique under operation room conditions
   c. Presterilized packaged components
   d. Antibiotic cover

2. **Minimize tissue injury by:**
   a. Gentle surgical technique
   b. Sharp disposable drills of increasing sizes
   c. Light and intermittent drilling pressure
   d. Controlled rotational drill speeds and controlled torque
   e. Copious cooling irrigation

3. **Avoid contamination of implant surfaces by:**
   a. Separating titanium and stainless steel components and instruments
   b. Using only titanium instruments to touch titanium components
   c. Maintaining sterile technique
   d. Not touching titanium implants with gloves, suction tubing, or anything other than titanium

# Surgical Considerations

The maintenance of asepsis and sterility is crucial during these surgical stages. All implant surgery should be performed with due regard for standard sterile operating technique and with antibiotic cover. Special care should be taken to avoid contamination of the integrating surfaces of the titanium components. The handling of the tissues should be as gentle as possible, and copious coolant should be used during all heat-generating steps. The removal of the bone should be incremental so as to minimize bony trauma. The drills should be sharp, and the drilling pressure should be light and intermittent.

The incision for implant placement is commonly made in the labial vestibule, away from the crest of the ridge, and a flap developed that is lingually or palatally based, so that the suture line does not directly overlie the implant sites. This is felt to minimize the risk of contamination of the implants from the oral cavity. In certain circumstances, a crestal incision may be preferred; for example, where the normal vascularity of the soft tissues has been already impaired by previous surgery.

When the implant system is of the single stage (nonsubmerged) type, the implant penetrates the mucosa immediately. In such cases it is felt wiser to avoid loading the implants until after a suitable healing period. The ITI system follows this pattern.

When implants are cylindrical without threads, the thread-tapping step is omitted from the site preparation; this implant type relies on "press-fit" friction for placement into the site. This applies to the IMZ and other cylindrical systems.

Regardless of which type of endosseous implant is used, the chances of successful osseointegration will be enhanced by adherence to certain points of surgical protocol designed to minimize tissue trauma, avoid contamination, maintain sterility, and maximize precision.

# Reference

1. Adell R, Lekholm U, Brånemark P-I. Surgical procedures. In: Brånemark P-I, Zarb GA, Albrektsson T (eds). Tissue-Integrated Prostheses: Osseointegration in Clinical Dentistry. Chicago: Quintessence, 1985: 211–232.

# 9

# Prosthodontic Aspects of Dental Implants

*Brien R. Lang*

Implant-supported prostheses have become an important therapy for partial and full edentulism. While there are many different implant types and designs, they all require a high degree of prosthodontic skill for success. The key to prosthodontic treatment success is a well-organized and well-performed data gathering process. Data gathered before treatment is used to select not only the appropriate implants and to determine the surgical protocols, but to define the nature of the prosthodontic therapy.

Securing dental casts of the patient and mounting these casts on a dental articulator will provide a great deal of information about the existing oral conditions that may not be apparent during the oral examination. The diagnostic mounting offers all clinicians involved the opportunity to design optimal occlusal contacts and to determine the need for additional restorative care.

Selection of the implant design for a patient can initially be made from the diagnostic mounting. Once the implant has been selected, the choice of surgical approach can be considered. A number of implant designs

## The Diagnostic Mounting

are available to the profession for use in restoring a missing tooth or teeth. The three most frequently used designs are the subperiosteal, transosseous, and endosseous implants. (For illustrations of these types of implants, see Chapter 1.) The diagnostic mounting can help the members of the implant team decide how many implants will be needed and the best positions for their placement in the bone. Determining the best implant or implants for clinical application depends on the existing oral conditions and the dimensions and location of the edentulous space to be treated.

### Subperiosteal Implants

These implants are individually designed cast-metal frames made from an impression and master cast of the anatomical site where the implant will be placed.[1,2] Metal posts project from the implant frame to penetrate the oral mucosa and enter the mouth. Support and retention of an implant prosthesis are provided by these posts.

The subperiosteal implant is cast in surgical vitallium, and is without special surface coatings or preparations. The implant frame rests on bone for support, and may or may not be fixed to the bone by screws.

Both short and long edentulous spans in the maxilla and mandible have been restored by this implant; however, it has been primarily used for the mandible of the completely edentulous patient.

### Transosseous Implants

These implants pass through bone.[3] The transosseous implant consists of a flat bone plate fitted to the lower border of the mandible. Projecting from the bone plate are a number of posts; some posts insert into the bone for retention, while other posts pass through the bone to penetrate the oral mucosa. Prosthetic attachments that fit the intraoral posts provide the means of prosthesis retention.[3]

Transosseous design variations relate to the number

of posts on the bone plate for retention, and the number that penetrate the oral cavity for prosthesis support. There are normally two or four posts for prosthesis retention, depending on the specific patient's prosthodontic needs.

Transosseous implants are machined from commercially pure titanium, a titanium alloy, or a gold alloy, unlike subperiosteal implants, which are cast. The surfaces of the posts are threaded, and special surface coatings or preparations are not customary.

## Endosseous Implants

Endosseous implants are positioned within the jaw bone and gain support from bone by osseointegration.[3] The implant designs are varied, yet generally conform to the shape of a natural tooth root. Some implants are designed as cylinders (Fig 9-1). Other implant forms are screws (Fig 9-2).

The endosseous implant is machined from commercially pure titanium or a titanium alloy, and is cleaned, sterilized, and packaged in a sterile container ready for use. The endosseous implant surface may be coated or sprayed to create a textured surface to potentially enhance osseointegration. More information is needed on the osseointegrative function of these surface preparations, as well as on their general biocompatibility.

Generally, endosseous implants have an intraosseous component surgically placed in the patient's maxilla or mandible, and called simply the implant (Fig 9-3a). This provides retention for the entire implant structure. A cover screw (Fig 9-3b) is used during initial healing.

The implant abutment cylinder, usually referred to simply as the abutment (Fig 9-3c), is joined to the implant fixture and penetrates the mucosa, entering the oral environment as the transmucosal component of the implant framework. The abutment is attached to the implant with the abutment screw (Fig 9-3d). The accurate orientation of these two components at their interface varies for each endosseous implant. In certain endosseous implants, the implant and abutment are

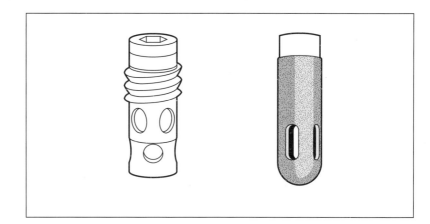

**Fig 9-1** Endosseous implants designed as cylinders.

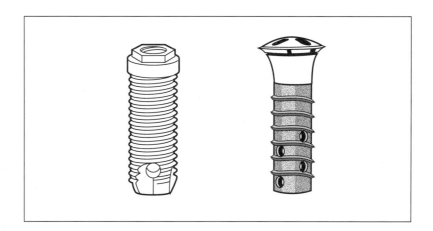

**Fig 9-2** Endosseous implants designed as screws.

designed as a single unit, eliminating the need for the abutment screw. These two components in combination represent the tooth root analog.

The third component in endosseous implants is similar to a post and core in conventional prosthodontics, which may be a single unit or two separate parts. For example, the core may be a gold or titanium cylinder (Figs 9-3e and f) joined to the abutment by a gold screw (Fig 9-3g) that represents the post. Located in the center of the abutment screw is a threaded opening that will accommodate the screw used to join the core to the abutment. For some single tooth implants, the core is incorporated into a wax pattern that is cast to form a framework on which porcelain is fused or artificial teeth processed

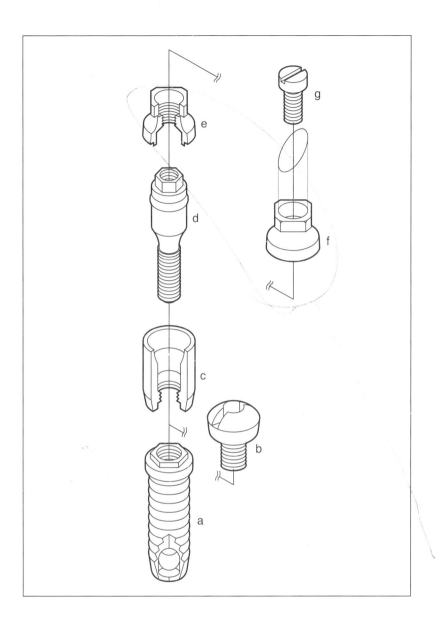

**Fig 9-3a–g**  Brånemark System components. *a:* implant; *b:* cover screw; *c:* abutment; *d:* abutment screw; *e, f:* cylinders; *g:* gold screw.

to produce the implant prosthesis. The finished crown is attached to the abutment by a gold screw (Fig 9-4). For some endosseous implants, the core is made from dense sintered aluminum oxide and offers optimal esthetics when combined with an outer layer of porcelain (Fig 9-5). In still other situations, the abutment is shaped to receive a replacement crown made and cemented to the abutment in the conventional manner (Fig 9-6). Machined titanium cores are also available that can be

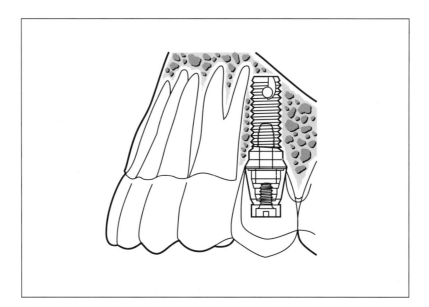

**Fig 9-4**   The implant core is incorporated into a cast crown, which is attached to the abutment by a gold screw.

laser-welded to other preformed titanium units to create an implant framework. Other cores are used as stand-alone units or cast in a framework design that is screwed to the abutments to provide support and retention for an overdenture (Figs 9-7a and b). With the endosseous implant, selection of the abutment and core design should be deferred until after surgery has been completed.

Regardless of design, endosseous implants are the basic tooth root analog units in implant prosthodontic protocols, and are by far the most frequently used implants for oral rehabilitation.

The diagnostic mounting can help initiate design of the implant prosthesis. The definitive prosthesis will differ depending on the location and dimensions of the edentulous space and on the success of implant placement. Single-tooth replacement, multiple-tooth spans in partially edentulous jaws, and the totally edentulous arch are the most frequent clinical situations treated with implants. The presence or absence of specific factors in each of these situations, as observed clinically and/or determined from the diagnostic mounting, contribute to determining the best implant design.

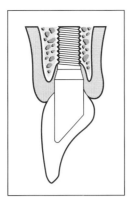
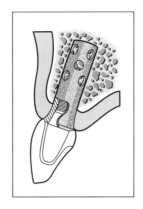

**Fig 9-5 *(left)*** The implant core is a dense sintered aluminum oxide that is combined with a layer of porcelain to create the crown restoration.

**Fig 9-6 *(right)*** The abutment may be a single unit screwed to the implant, with the crown cemented directly to it.

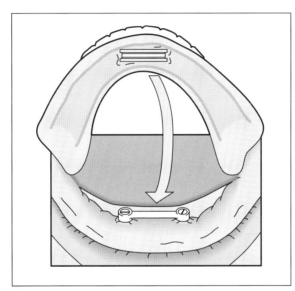

**Fig 9-7a** Implants can be joined by nonflexible bars, which are used with resilient bar attachments. These implant frameworks provide excellent retention for overdentures.

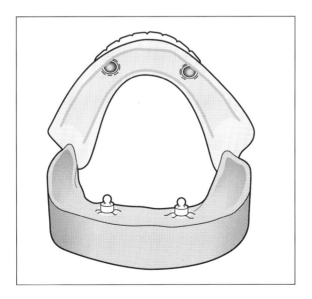

**Fig 9-7b** Implants can also be used as single units, with ball attachments to provide overdenture retention. The use of spacers and rubber O-rings allows rotation around the ball, while the posterior supporting mandibular areas restrict tilting.

## Single-Tooth Implants

The amount of space between the teeth adjacent to the edentulous area is critical to the success of the single tooth implant.[4] A space that is too wide will not produce the desired esthetic results. A space that is too narrow to accommodate the implant may be widened by orthodontic therapy. If this will not improve the situation, then other prosthodontic options may be considered.

The contour of the ridge in the edentulous site is equally important. If the bone height is inadequate, it will be difficult to achieve the contour profiles between the implant and the supporting bone normally present at the junction of a natural tooth with its supporting tissues. Bone grafting or guided tissue regeneration procedures are techniques that can greatly improve these bone and soft tissue contours.

The position of the free gingival tissues on the proximal surfaces of the adjacent teeth is an important consideration in planning the single-tooth implant restoration. The prosthesis should be designed to provide for the maintenance of the tissue as interdental papillae and thereby achieve a natural-looking restoration.

## Multiple-Tooth Spans In Partially Edentulous Arches

When more than one tooth is to be restored, the size of the edentulous area and the amount of bone available for implant placement will influence the number of implants to be placed. In the partially edentulous situations, two or more implants is the norm (Fig 9-8).

The location of the implants is important to prosthesis design. Arranging artificial teeth or using wax to contour anticipated replacement teeth for the edentulous area is a common practice with the diagnostic mounting. This approach will also determine how the prosthetic replacement teeth will meet the occlusal demands in rehabilitation. After the diagnostic arrangement of the artificial teeth is completed, the proposed locations for the implants can be decided. Generally, the implant

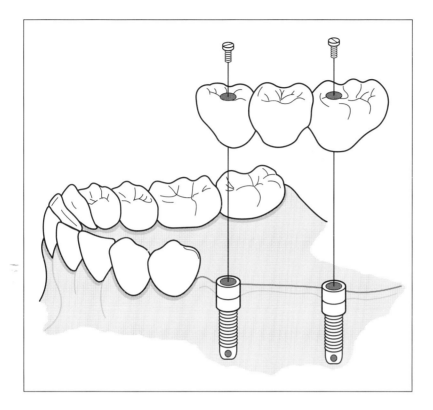

**Fig 9-8**  The location of implants is important to the design of the multiple-tooth prosthesis. Generally, the implants should be positioned so that the core component can be centered in a tooth within the prosthesis.

should be positioned so that the core component can be centered in a tooth in the prosthesis. In some situations this may not be possible, because there may not be enough bone available in the location selected to support the implant.

## Totally Edentulous Maxillary and Mandibular Arches

The diagnostic mounting is often considered unnecessary with the totally edentulous patient. However, failure to use such a mounting may result in a prosthesis design compromise during treatment that might have been foreseen and avoided through the study of a diagnostic mounting. The diagnostic mounting for the edentulous patient is considerably different from the mounting for the partially edentulous patient. In some instances it will be necessary to duplicate the patient's existing dentures, while other situations demand a new denture as a diagnostic device to plan the implant placement and final prosthesis design.

# Stage I Surgery: Prosthodontic Procedures

The use of a diagnostic mounting is invaluable in projecting the goal of treatment, regardless of whether a single implant or a number of implants are to be placed. During treatment planning, mounted casts are essential for diagnosis and for the fabrication of implant positioning devices. Implants in poor positions are as much the responsibility of the restorative dentist as they are of the surgeon who placed the implants. Without an adequate presurgical work-up and the preparation of surgical positioning devices or guides, surgeons cannot be expected to place implants in sites useful for prosthetic reconstruction. Acrylic templates are easy to fabricate and can make surgical procedures much more effective. There are a number of techniques that are published elsewhere for making guides or stents.[5]

It is ideal for the dentist to be present during surgery to assist the surgeon in the decision-making process, even when surgical guides are available. When it is discovered, for example, that inadequate bone exists at the implant site originally planned, the entire implant team should be available to discuss possible modifications to implant placement, prosthesis design, and surgical guides.

Provisional restorations following Stage I surgery are essential for many patients, as they simply cannot go without their teeth. For totally edentulous implant patients, any contact with the surgical site by a provisional denture during the first 10 to 14 days following Stage I surgery may prove quite uncomfortable and therefore must be delayed. If the provisional denture is worn too early, the osseointegration rate will decrease. As soon as it is practical, however, the provisional denture should be placed and maintained for the duration of the healing period. A soft denture-base reline material should be used to adapt the denture base to the healing tissue sites (Fig 9-9). It is still important during this

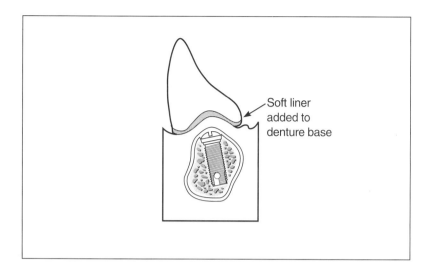

Soft liner
added to
denture base

**Fig 9-9**  Following Stage I surgery, a patient's existing denture can be relined with a soft denture-base material to serve as a provisional restoration during the 4 to 5 months of postoperative healing.

entire healing phase not to load the implants directly. All borders of the provisional denture must be shortened and an adequate thickness of soft liner added.

The patient may have questions and concerns, and may need encouragement while waiting to find out if the implants are indeed integrating with the bone. This waiting period may be very stressful for some patients, and any change in their oral status may cause concern. Replacing the soft lining material several times during the months following Stage I surgery will do more than just keep the material in good condition; it will show the dentist's concern for the patient.

Once the implant is brought into the oral cavity by placement of the abutments during Stage II surgery, it is important to reemphasize the oral hygiene regimen so that the tissues around the biocompatible surfaces develop healthily. For some patients, hygiene will include chemical agents in addition to the mechanical plaque removal recommended for all patients. During the approximately 2 weeks of healing following Stage II surgery, the provisional dentures may greatly assist in the healing process by positioning the tissues for future

# Stage II Surgery: Prosthodontic Procedures

prosthetic considerations. Modifications to the tissue surface of the denture base by removal of some acrylic resin and the previously placed soft liner will permit seating of the denture over the abutments that now extend into the mouth. When adequate clearance has been created in the denture base to accommodate the abutments, a new application of the soft liner can be placed. This helps to position the healing mucosal tissues around the abutments. Once tissues around the abutments begin to show signs of a favorable color response and manipulations of the tissues in the area can be performed without discomfort, the definitive reconstruction procedures can begin. It is important to explain to the patient that following Stage II surgery there is no period when the existing prosthesis cannot be worn. During the remaining prosthodontic procedures and up to completion of the treatment plan, the patient may continue to function with the existing prosthesis.

If the treatment plan involves a partially edentulous area and a single- or multiple-implant restoration, the initial abutments placed are usually healing abutments, with final abutment selection delayed until later. With the wide array of esthetic abutment choices, a tissue healing period is needed to determine the most advantageous abutment for the particular reconstructive plan. Once the abutment has been selected, a variety of temporary components are available for use in fabricating a provisional partial denture or single-tooth replacement while definitive prosthodontic treatment is underway.

# Definitive Prosthodontic Treatment

Continued long-term success with implant therapy can be expected as long as surgical and prosthetic procedures are adjusted to the anatomy, healing potential, hard and soft tissue remodeling capacity, and maintenance capabilities of the patient.[6-8] Generally, the prognosis for implants in partially edentulous patients has been approximately the same as corresponding treatment for totally edentulous patients. There does not seem to be any advantage to connecting natural teeth and implant abutments in the same fixed implant-supported applications. In fact, a more favorable situation is present when the biomechanically different tooth-supported and implant-supported prosthetic applications are kept as separate units. The use of a tissue-integrated prosthesis presents a wider range of complex technical and biological problems in the partially edentulous patient than in the completely edentulous patient. In the totally edentulous maxilla or mandible, the replacement of the lost dentition can be accomplished using either the implant-supported fixed prosthesis or the implant-supported overdenture. Treatment for the partially edentulous patient is more technically demanding and varied than it is for patients with no remaining natural teeth.

The basic prosthodontic treatment protocols for implant therapy include single-tooth implants, multiple-tooth replacements in partially edentulous jaws, and restoration of the totally edentulous maxilla and mandible. Each treatment protocol has differences or variations in technique for impression making, registration of maxillomandibular jaw relations, implant framework design, and occlusal considerations. Because there are numerous publications that present in great detail each step in the treatment protocols,[4–12] only those aspects of prosthodontic treatment that are uniquely different from conventional prosthodontics in restoring similar tooth loss situations will be discussed.

## Single-Tooth Implants

The single-tooth implant is especially appropriate in the anterior maxilla of young patients with otherwise intact dentitions. Conventional treatment using a three-unit prosthesis or a removable partial denture may be more appropriate in situations where caries, periodontal support, and lack of space for an implant exist.[11]

Perhaps the most compelling reason for single-tooth implant replacements is the required sacrifice of healthy tooth substance from adjacent teeth with the conventional three-unit fixed prosthesis. The principal indication for treatment with the single-tooth implant occurs in anterior and premolar areas in which the neighboring teeth are unsuitable for preparation as abutments for a conventional fixed prosthesis. The single-implant restoration is the treatment of choice if the patient's esthetic expectations are realistic.

Pronounced bruxism, a short lip, and local vertical resorption of the alveolar process are factors that would compromise the use of the single-tooth implant.

If the implant is positioned appropriately, then the normal restorative procedures for the single-tooth implant can proceed. However, if the implant is malaligned, then it will be necessary before proceeding to use one of the innovative prosthetic devices that have been developed to correct the alignment (Fig 9-10).

Where the space available is adequate and the ridge contours are acceptable, the abutment selection is relatively easy. Abutment components are available in several lengths to accommodate the thickness of the mucosa over the bone (Fig 9-11). The variations in length also provide a means of controlling the placement of the margins of the final implant restoration in relation to the gingiva. In the anterior maxillary region, the shorter abutments are most commonly used. With these shorter units, the restoration margins can be placed subgingivally to satisfy most esthetic requirements.

The decisions regarding the implant core design and whether the prosthesis will be cemented or screwed to the abutment should be made before the initiation of definitive treatment.

The impression procedure for the single-tooth implant is quite different from the impression technique used in conventional prosthodontics for a prepared natural tooth. With implants, the impression is made using an impression coping screwed or pressed into place on the abutment. The impression materials, tray design, and technique will vary depending on the coping selected. In any case, the impression coping becomes part of the impression. Once the impression is made, a replica of the abutment is screwed or pressed to the coping and the dental cast is poured in improved stone.

In most techniques, the impression material is syringed around the impression coping, and the impres-

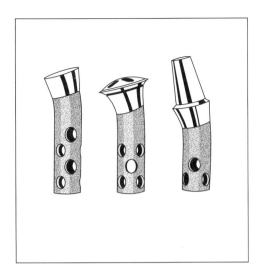

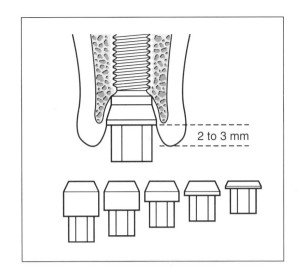

sion tray is seated over the coping. The impression is removed from the mouth, and a replica is connected to the impression coping. Before preparing the master cast, a plasticized acrylic material can be poured around the neck of the coping to create the gingival margins in a soft material. The remainder of the cast is poured in improved stone.

Record bases may or may not be necessary to make the appropriate maxillomandibular records. In any case, the master casts for the maxilla and mandible are mounted on the dental articulator in the maximum intercuspal position.

The core pattern for the definitive restoration is completed incorporating the material selected for the implant prosthesis. Both resin-to-metal and porcelain-to-metal constructions have been used. All porcelain restorations using a sintered aluminum oxide have shown excellent esthetic results. If a metal casting is to be used, it must be evaluated intraorally before completing the restoration. The implant metal framework must seat completely and passively on the abutments, and any discrepancy requires a remake of the framework.

It appears desirable, particularly when the implant restoration is in the maxilla, for the natural dentition to provide anterior guidance during lateral excursion. Posterior implants should maintain occlusal contact in

**Fig 9-10** *(left)*   Abutment specifically designed to correct for malalignment by adjusting the final angle of the artificial tooth crown.

**Fig 9-11** *(right)*   Abutment components are available in several lengths to meet the individual needs of different implant sites. The height of the abutment should be 2 to 3 mm less than the distance between the gingival margin and the head of the implant.

maximum intercuspation. It is recommended that if adequate anterior guidance with the natural dentition exists, the implant-supported restoration should be free of contacts with the opposing dentition during lateral and protrusive jaw movement.

## Multiple-Tooth Replacements In Partially Edentulous Arches

Dental implants are used as abutments for multiple-tooth replacements in partially edentulous situations in the anterior and posterior parts of the maxilla and mandible. A missing premolar and molar in the maxillary arch is a good example. In the maxillary anterior region, shorter abutments are the more commonly used component (Fig 9-12). In partially edentulous posterior situations, longer abutments are the more common choice because they provide greater access for oral hygiene procedures.

For most partially edentulous situations, the prosthesis design incorporates an implant core component that screws to the abutment and permits retrieval of the prosthesis for cleaning and maintenance. The core component may have metal cast to it or it may come as a

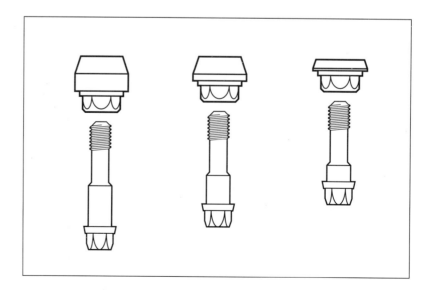

**Fig 9-12**    Different lengths of titanium collars allow flexibility in the termination point of the final implant structure.

unified part of a laser-welded titanium framework. This latter framework has the additional advantage of using titanium throughout the construction.

Making impressions of the existing oral conditions and accurately registering the abutments in multiple-tooth replacement situations are similar to the techniques used with the single-tooth implant. Various forms of tapered and square copings are used in impression making; however, great care must be exercised in registering the spatial relationships between the abutments. The pouring of the master cast from the final impression differs little from the technique previously described. Regardless of the technique used to create the master cast, its verification for accuracy and replication of the oral conditions is of paramount importance to the success of treatment.

Using a verification index can ensure that these positional and spatial relationships have been recorded in the impression and transferred to the master cast (Fig 9-13). The coping used to make the impression is the component most often used to make a verification index. After the copings have been fitted to their analogs in the master cast, they are bonded as a unit using a chemically or light-activated acrylic resin. The implant copings must fit the abutment surfaces accurately and passively to assure a precision fit at their interface during index construction.

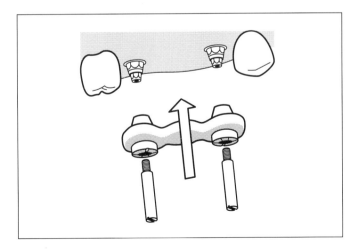

**Fig 9-13**   A verification index is fitted to the analogs of the implants on the master cast to check alignment.

The verification index must fit the abutment replicas on the master cast and the abutments in the mouth in the same relationship. Using the index, one is able to determine if the master cast is accurate, and to confirm that the correct spatial relations of the implant abutments have been recorded and transferred from the mouth to the master cast. The detailed steps in fabrication of the verification index are described in other texts and will not be presented here; their importance in implant-based prosthodontics, however, cannot be overemphasized.

Record bases are usually necessary in the partially edentulous situation to record and transfer the appropriate maxillomandibular records from the patient to the articulator. Incorporating the core component in the record base will increase stability and provide the retention to assure accurate registration and transfer. The master casts are mounted on the dental articulator in the maximum intercuspal position.

The wax pattern for the definitive restoration is prepared by incorporating the implant core selected for the patient into the framework design. The pattern design is influenced by the materials to be used in the final restoration. The pattern for a porcelain-to-metal restoration is similar to that used for traditional fixed prosthodontics and, as always, the metal casting is evaluated intraorally before completing the restoration. The implant metal framework must seat completely and passively. Any discrepancy will require the framework to be sectioned, a new relationship secured, and the framework reunited. When a precise fit is attained, the restoration can be finished by the addition of the desired esthetic material.

If artificial teeth are to be added to the implant framework, a means of retention must be either developed in the wax pattern or chemically added to the completed framework. When porcelain is used to restore function, form, and esthetics, the appropriate supporting surface must be developed in the framework wax pattern. Artificial teeth are added to the laser-welded framework in the manner previously described. A unique porcelain that fuses at low temperatures is used for application to titanium framework.

For the multiple-tooth implant that is not replacing the canine, the occlusal considerations are similar to those encountered in the normal course of providing fixed partial denture services. Canine-guided or mutually protected schemes release the implant prosthesis from laterally directed forces. The group-function occlusal scheme (multiple working side contacts in lateral excursions) is equally appropriate, especially for those patients in whom implants have been used to replace more than a single tooth, which calls for the distribution of forces over several implants.

### Totally Edentulous Maxillary and Mandibular Arches

The ideal oral rehabilitation of the totally edentulous arch is a fixed implant-supported prosthesis (Fig 9-14). Patients who have been provided this service have

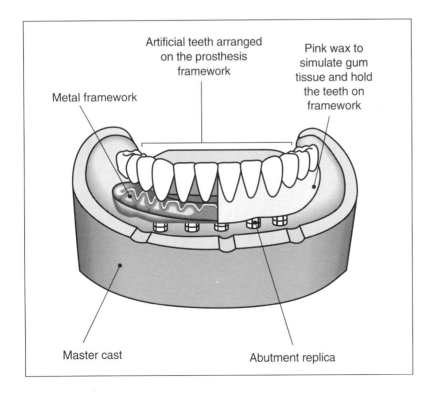

**Fig 9-14**  A master cast showing the prosthodontic simulation of a fixed implant-supported prosthesis for an totally edentulous mandible.

reported satisfaction with function and comfort. However, this approach is not always possible. There are anatomical and functional limitations present in some patients that preclude the use of a fixed prosthesis. However, the predominant reason for selecting an overdenture instead of a fixed prosthesis is economic.

If the loss of the natural teeth and the alveolar bone associated with their support creates severe anatomical deficiencies, then the treatment protocol of choice is an implant-supported overdenture. If the bone quantity and quality available limits the surgeon to placing only two or three implants, then an overdenture is also indicated. If four or more implants can be positioned appropriately, and the anatomic features of bone loss and alveolar support are not limiting factors, then a fixed prosthesis is the restoration of choice.

Esthetic and phonetic concerns are problems associated with severe resorption and tooth loss. Restoring the lost bulk associated with the supporting alveolus by a fixed prosthesis is often impossible; however, these anatomical features can be restored with an implant-supported overdenture, thereby avoiding esthetic and phonetic problems associated with the loss of these tissues.

If oral hygienic maintenance will be compromised by complex designs in reconstruction using a fixed prosthesis, then an overdenture is the treatment of choice.

Patients with jaw defects or unusual jaw relations that would create adverse biomechanical conditions with a fixed prosthesis should instead receive an implant-supported overdenture reconstruction.[12]

Implants are most often placed in the mandibular arch; however, this does not mean that an implant prosthesis in the maxillary arch is unnecessary or undesirable. Most edentulous patients are able to wear a conventional maxillary complete denture with reasonable success. However, for patients with extremely resorbed maxillary ridges or other anatomic considerations that preclude successful denture wearing, the implant-supported prosthesis is an excellent treatment option. The retention achieved with a conventional maxillary denture is not acceptable to some patients, and implants have been suggested for improved retention in these cases.

The restoration of the totally edentulous mandibular arch requires that access be provided for cleaning the abutments. In this situation, a lesser concern for esthetics has also resulted in the longer abutment becoming the more frequently used component. Again, the appropriate abutment selection must be completed before definitive treatment is initiated.

Impression of the edentulous arch and the accurate registration of the spatial relationships of the abutments is similar to the technique used with multiple-tooth replacements. The preliminary impression is made with irreversible hydrocolloid with the tapered coping in place on the abutments (Fig 9-15). The copings are removed from the mouth and connected to the brass analogs. The entire assembly is inserted into the impression and a preliminary cast is poured in improved stone. The square copings are used for the master cast impression. Their design allows them to become locked into the impression material (Fig 9-16). This impression cannot be removed from the oral cavity unless the guide screws used to hold the copings in position are loosened and removed from the mouth.

Customized impression trays are made prior to the impression procedure; their design is determined by the choice of a fixed implant-supported prosthesis or an implant-supported overdenture. In the latter situation, the impression tray is usually designed for complete

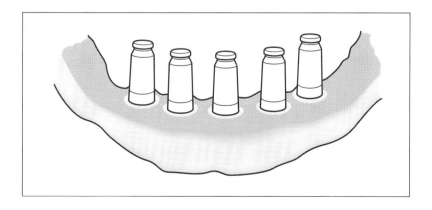

**Fig 9-15**   Tapered copings screwed to the abutments.

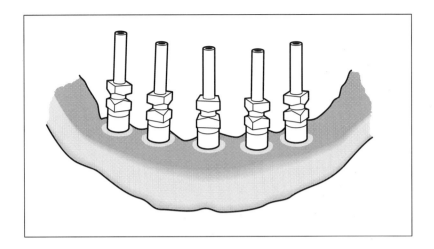

**Fig 9-16** Square impression copings are used to make the final impression. These copings are usually joined using a chemically activated acrylic resin, maintaining their spatial relationships during impression-making.

border molding, similar to impression-making for a conventional denture. The tray for a fixed implant-supported prosthesis does not require these border extensions, and need only extend to record the primary residual ridge and retromolar pads, since they are important landmarks in determining the occlusal plane location in the final restoration. In both trays, a relief space is required in the area of the copings to provide for a sufficient thickness of impression material around the impression copings. Before making the final impression, the square impression copings must be accurately seated on their respective abutments, and then luted together using an acrylic resin material. The final impression is made using any number of the impression materials available. The master cast is poured in improved dental stone.

The verification index is used to ensure the accurate replication of the oral conditions, so that the positional relationships of the abutments are correctly recorded in the impression and transferred to the master cast.

Accurate, stable, and retentive record bases are required in the totally edentulous situation to record and transfer the appropriate maxillomandibular records from the patient to the articulator. Incorporating the core component within the record base increases stability and provides the retention necessary to assure accurate registration and transfer. The design of the record base is similar to the extension and form used in conventional complete denture prosthodontics. The master casts are mounted on the dental articulator in the centric relation jaw position. The vertical dimension of occlusion and centric relation transferred to the articulator must also be verified by a second interocclusal record. A protrusive record is also needed to set the condylar elements of the articulator to the degree mechanical equivalents simluating the horizontal shape of the patient's condylar eminence before arranging the replacement teeth on the record base.

Selection and arrangement of the artificial teeth is usually completed before construction of the implant framework, regardless of whether the prosthesis is a fixed implant-supported type or an implant-supported overdenture. There are tooth designs, developed specifically for implant patients, that maximize control over the direction of force applications, which is of vital importance. Whenever possible, these designs should be used.[13] The principles for arranging teeth are based on a lingualized articulation. For this arrangement there are a number of factors that can influence the positioning of the artificial teeth in the dental arch. One of these factors is the incisal guidance, or the amount of vertical and horizontal overlap of the maxillary anterior teeth over the mandibular anterior teeth. Minimizing the vertical overlap and maximizing the horizontal overlap within the limitations of an acceptable esthetic result will reduce the occlusal forces to the anterior residual ridge. The positioning of the occlusal surfaces of the lower artifical teeth in relation to the corners of the mouth and the retromolar pads in an anteroposterior relation provides the appropriate occlusal plane for mastication and distribution of the forces from function. The buccolingual placement of the lower artificial teeth in relation to the crest of the residual ridge assures the proper arch arrangement for interdigitation of the mandibular teeth with their maxillary antagonists. Finally, the orientation of the mandibular teeth with their cusps arranged to anteroposterior and mediolateral compensating curves assures that the contacts of the opposing maxillary teeth will be smooth and free-gliding during movements of the mandible into lateral positions.

The pattern design for the implant framework is established after the teeth have been arranged and the clinical try-in completed. A cast or laser-welded framework construction is usually employed. A silicone-putty tooth index, keyed to the master cast, provides the technician with the needed information to fabricate the framework. This index allows determination of the available space between the teeth and the implant cores, where the framework will be formed. It is important that at least 2 to 3 mm of space exists between the soft tissues and the undersurface of the implant-supported framework. A space of less than 2 mm makes it difficult for patients to maintain an acceptable level of oral hygiene. The contour of the tissue surface of the framework should be convex to facilitate cleansing, and the facial-lingual dimension of the prosthesis must be kept minimal to facilitate access for oral hygiene.

If the prosthesis is to be implant-supported, then elements of the framework design must be incorporated that will provide a means of attaching the replacement teeth and the supporting acrylic resin to the framework. If the framework is to support an overdenture, then a number of other retention mechanisms are available that can be incorporated into the framework wax pattern.

The metal framework should be evaluated intraorally, both by visual and radiographic examination, before completing the restoration. Accurate fit at the prosthodontic interface between the framework and the abutments is crucial to the biomechanics of the implant-supported prosthesis. If the elements are malaligned, the magnitude and direction of forces transferred from activities like chewing may exceed the tolerable limits at the implant-bone interface. An overlooked gap between the abutments and the prosthesis, for example, could produce uneven force distribution, which could negatively affect the lifetime survival rate of the implants. If malalignment is observed, either visually or radiographically, the problem must be corrected before proceeding with any further prosthodontic procedure.

Research reports have demonstrated that forces generated by patients with implants during maximum occlusion have approached the forces registered by patients with natural dentitions. In some instances maximum occlusal forces have been recorded for implant patients that exceed the normal force for the dentate patient.[14,15] Therefore, in a totally edentulous implant patient whose implant-supported prosthesis involves the full arch and opposes an artificial dentition, it is essential that an occlusal scheme be used that is capable of distributing occlusal forces evenly over the entire opposing arch and equally to each abutment. Bilateral balance and the concept of lingualized articulation are suggested, because the tooth forms associated with this occlusal scheme require less occlusal force to achieve mastication and there are no deflective occlusal contacts in the various jaw movements.[13]

Processing and finishing of the implant restorations are somewhat different than these same procedures carried out on conventional fixed or removable prostheses. Information regarding the techniques can be found in the previously cited implant texts.

# References

1.  Perel ML. Dental Implantology and Prostheses. Philadelphia: Lippincott, 1977:1–49.

2.  Taylor TD, Laney WR. Dental Implants: Are They For Me? Chicago: Quintessence, 1990.

3.  Beumer J III, Lewis SG. The Brånemark Implant System: clinical laboratory procedures. St Louis: Ishiyau EuroAmerica, 1989:31–37, 157–167.

4.  Parel SM, Lewis S. The Smiline System. Dallas: Taylor Publishing Company, 1991:9–11.

5.  Brånemark P-I. Introduction to osseointegration. In: Brånemark P-I, Zarb GA, Albrektsson T (eds). Tissue-Integrated Prostheses: Osseointegration in Clinical Dentistry. Chicago: Quintessence, 1985:155–198.

6.  Lekholm U, Torsten J. Principles for single tooth replacement. In: Albrektsson T, Zarb GA (eds). The Brånemark Osseointegrated Implant. Chicago: Quintessence, 1989:117–126.

7.  van Steenberghe D. The impact of osseointegrated prostheses on treatment planning in oral rehabilitation. In: Albrektsson T, Zarb

GA (eds). The Brånemark Osseointegrated Implant. Chicago: Quintessence, 1989:139–145.

8. Laney WR, Tolman, DE. The Mayo Clinic experience with tissue-integrated prostheses. In: Albrektsson T, Zarb GA (eds). The Brånemark Osseointegrated Implant. Chicago: Quintessence, 1989:165–195.

9. Hobo S, Ichida E, Garcia LT. Osseointegration and Occlusal Rehabilitation. Chicago: Quintessence, 1989:65–73.

10. Ericsson I, Brånemark P-I, Glantz P-O. Partial edentulism. In: Worthington P, Brånemark P-I (eds). Advanced Osseointegration Surgery: Applications in the Maxillofacial Region. Chicago: Quintessence, 1992:194–209.

11. Ohrnell L-O, Palmquist J, Brånemark P-I. Single tooth replacement. In: Worthington P, Brånemark P-I (eds). Advanced Osseointegration Surgery: Applications in the Maxillofacial Region. Chicago: Quintessence, 1992:194–209.

12. Engquist B. Overdentures. In: Worthington P, Brånemark P-I (eds). Advanced Osseointegration Surgery: Applications in the Maxillofacial Region. Chicago: Ouintessence 1992:233–247.

13. Lang BR, Razzoog ME. Lingualized integration: Tooth molds and an occlusal scheme for edentulous implant patients. Implant Dent 1992;204–211.

14. Haraldson T, Zarb GA. 10-year follow-up study of the masticatory system after treatment with osseointegrated implant bridges. Scand J Dent Res 1988;24–52.

15. Michael CG, Javid NS, Colaizzi FA, Gibbs CH. Biting strength and chewing forces in complete denture wearers. J Prosthet Dent 1990;63:549–553.

# 10

# Maintenance

*Michael E. Razzoog*

There are four elements in the maintenance program for the patient with dental implants. First is the establishment of a home-care regimen in personal oral hygiene that helps the patient achieve an acceptable level of plaque control. The second element is reinforcement of this regimen by periodic recall appointments, which evaluate the patient's progress and monitor the status of the implants and the health of the supporting tissues. Strict adherence to a recall schedule and verifying that the implant prosthesis continues to satisfy the requirements of function, comfort, and esthetics initially established is the third element in the maintenance program. The fourth element is a lifetime commitment by the patient to the tenets of the maintenance program; this is the overriding factor in long-term prosthetic implant success.

Meticulous home care must be demonstrated by the patient during the presurgical phase of treatment. To insure good oral hygiene, the daily home-care program of the patient must be customized to the individual's ability

## A Home-Care Regimen in Oral Hygiene

to keep plaque off the remaining natural teeth. Emphasis must be directed toward the proper use of a tooth brush, and the use of dental floss to clean debris from around the remaining natural teeth.[1,2]

After placement of the implants in Stage I surgery, hygiene recall visits at appropriate intervals will be needed to continue the monitoring of plaque control, and to prevent the occurrence of an inflammatory response in the tissues around the natural teeth and in the area of the implants.

Uncovering the implants and placing the abutment components during Stage II surgery necessitates additional home-care considerations. The sutures used in the tissues adjacent to the abutment make it somewhat difficult to maintain oral hygiene. There is the tendency for patients to be afraid of damaging their implants and thus to be less aggressive in oral hygiene measures than is necessary. Additional instruction in oral hygiene techniques with soft toothbrushes and end-tufted brushes can help patients keep the implant abutments clean. A number of interdental devices, including specialized flossing materials and oral irrigation devices, have been designed for cleaning the interproximal areas of teeth. If available, these devices should be used on both the natural teeth and the abutment surfaces, where they have proven equally beneficial in removing plaque.

Chlorhexidine, an antimicrobial agent, may be prescribed as an oral rinse to reduce the adherence of plaque to the surface of the implant abutment. However, rinsing must stop when the implant prosthesis is attached to the abutment because the solution will stain the artificial teeth and base materials of the prosthesis.[3] Instead, the chlorhexidine should be applied around the abutments with a brush or cotton-tipped swab to minimize staining and maximize the concentration of the agent at the soft tissue–abutment interface.

Regardless of the technique or device that is used by the patient in customizing the home-care program, plaque removal from teeth and the implant abutments is the ultimate goal.

Reinforcing the home-care program by periodic recall appointments to evaluate the status of the implants and the health of the supporting tissues is essential to the success of implant treatment. A recall appointment schedule must be set up following placement of the prosthesis and completion of the initial phases of prosthodontic treatment.

During the first year following the placement of the implant prosthesis, the patient should be seen every 3 to 4 months. After the first year, the patient should be placed on a recall schedule which meets the individual's needs; however, 6 months between recall appointments should be the longest interval considered for the patient with dental implants.

At each recall appointment, the dentist must assess the tissue surrounding the implant abutment. The dentist should consider any deviation in color and consistency from the state of health routinely observed about a sound implant abutment. In addition, spontaneous bleeding or bleeding induced by a toothbrush must be recorded in the patient's chart. Tissue surrounding the implant should appear light pink or coral in color, and be firm and resilient. Marginal gingiva around the abutment will usually taper to a knife-edge junction next to the abutment or the implant restoration. Probing of pocket depth, a commonly accepted measurement in the monitoring of the health of the periodontium around natural teeth, is sometimes used to evaluate the tissue-abutment interface. If a probe is to be used, it must be made of plastic to protect the abutment from being scratched.

The overall success of dental rehabilitation with an implant-supported prosthesis depends on continuous stability of the prosthesis, which in turn depends on the long-term anchorage of the individual implants. The maintenance of osseointegration along the entire

# Reinforcing Home Care at the Recall Appointment

# Status of the Implants at the Recall Appointment

implant surface and of marginal bone height along the vertical extent of the implant are the two factors necessary for proper implant anchorage. Both of these factors depend on local stress concentrations; the marginal bone height is also influenced by reactions in the marginal soft tissues around the implant.

Even distribution of stress among all the implants will contribute favorably to the maintenance of marginal bone close to the implants. The accuracy of fit of the prosthesis to the implants should be checked at recall examinations. Undue or uneven forces on the bone may lead to microfractures that could elicit the development of nonmineralized connective tissue. Optimizing stress distribution is of continuing importance in implant prosthodontics.

Some bone loss will be noted at recall examinations. Reports in the literature suggest that 1 to 1.5 mm of marginal bone is lost during the first year after prosthesis connection to the implants, mainly in response to the surgical trauma.[4] Subsequent annual marginal bone loss after the first year is around 0.05 to 0.1 mm. Therefore, a bone loss of less than 0.1 mm per year appears to be routine. This represents a loss of about 2 mm vertical bone support during the first 10 years following implant placement.

The 1978 Harvard Conference on dental implants concluded that implant survival rates in maxillae and mandibles were approximately 95% and 85%, respectively.[5] It would appear that it is more difficult to achieve and maintain osseointegration in maxillae than in mandibles. It was also reported that the majority of implant losses occur during the first year. Recall examinations are thus extremely important for ensuring the long-term success of osseointegrated implants.

## Oral Prophylaxis for the Implant Patient

Certain modifications in oral prophylactic procedures involving osseointegrated dental implants are necessary during recall appointments. Conventional metal instruments and ultrasonic cleaning devices may scratch the titanium components and/or loosen retention screws.[6] Plastic cleaning instruments that conform to the implant surface when properly positioned by the operator and that prevent abrasion of the implant abutment should be used instead.

For those situations in which calculus cannot be removed with plastic instruments, the careful use of an air-powder abrasive system may be indicated. Several of these machines are available, and although expensive, they are valuable in the removal of calculus from inaccessible places.

**Radiographic Monitoring**

Radiographs allow assessment of the implant-bone interface. No radiolucency should be evident around the implant in the bone. Healthy, stable implants will display normal trabecular bone in close contact with the implant surface. It is suggested that radiographs be taken every 3 months after initial placement of the implant. After the first year, radiographs should be taken once every 12 months.

# Status of the Implant Prosthesis at the Recall Appointment

The conditions most frequently seen during periodic recall appointments which require attention are gingivitis, soft tissue hyperplasia, small fistulae, exposed implant threads, fracture of the abutment screw, fracture of the anchorage mechanism between the prosthesis and the abutment, loss of optimal occlusal contacts, and fracture of the prosthodontic framework.

Loosening of implant components is the most frequently encountered condition, which underlines the importance of accurate fit between implant components, especially at the prosthodontic interface. Tightening the screws will temporarily correct the condition; however, should the condition recur, careful attention should be given to the accuracy of fit. Fracture of the abutment screw, fracture of the gold screw, and late loss of the implant are rare occurrences, but they also may be related to lack of precision of fit between the implant components and the prosthesis.

If the components are not loose and the patient is demonstrating reasonable oral hygiene, then no obvious advantage can be gained from the removal of the pros- thesis. However, the oral condition may be such that removal of the prosthesis is necessary to clean around the abutments. Most implant components from different manufacturers are not interchangeable, so the dentist must have on hand the appropriate components and instrumentation for the implant system used for the patient.

Cleaning the removed prosthesis is easily accom- plished using an ultrasonic cleaning device. If the pros- thesis requires instrumentation to remove tenacious calculus or to polish the metal surfaces, the metal com- ponents at the prosthodontic interface must be covered with laboratory protective caps or brass analogs. All den- tal personnel must exercise the greatest of care when cleaning these areas with instruments and polishing agents to avoid damage to the prosthodontic interface.

With the prosthesis removed, the abutment should be examined for looseness and tightened, if necessary, using the appropriate instrumentation. Experience has shown that loose abutment screws are responsible for most of the adverse tissue responses surrounding the abutment at recall appointments, including hyperplasia, hypertro- phy, and progressive marginal bone loss.

There should be no space at the prosthodontic inter- face. If a space is seen, the exact cause for the change must be pursued and corrected. Simply replacing the prosthesis and tightening the screws will ultimately lead to further complications and possible implant loss.

Excess forces resulting from malocclusion may also contribute to the early loss of an implant. At every recall appointment the restorative dentist must evaluate the occlusal contacts in centric and eccentric positions, look- ing for changes that have occurred due to wear or other factors. If corrections are necessary, they must be per- formed.

To prevent complications with dental implant treatment, the dentist must establish a healthy oral environment and the patient must aid in long-term implant maintenance. The patient must become a co-therapist and take a level of responsibility for his or her oral condition. This chapter has recommended a series of recall activities and strict protocols that have proven to be successful in promoting a continuous level of health. While these mechanisms are known to be helpful, the implant patient must be educated, and encouraged to understand his or her role in the maintenance of implant health.

# A Lifetime Commitment to Maintenance

# References

1.  Beumer J III, Lewis SG. The Brånemark Implant System: Clinical and Laboratory Procedures. St Louis: Ishiyau EuroAmerica, 1989:34–35, 100–103.

2.  Hobo S, Ichida E, Garcia LT. Osseointegration and Occlusal Rehabilitation. Chicago: Quintessence, 1989:239–254.

3.  Khokhar Z, Razzoog ME, Yaman P. Color stability of restorative resins. Quintessence Int 1991;22:733–737.

4.  Adell R, Lekholm U, Rockler B, Brånemark PI. A 15-year study of osseointegrated implants in the treatment of the edentulous jaw. Int J Oral Surg 1987;10:387–416.

5.  Schnitman PA, Shulman LB. Recommendations on the consensus development conference on dental implants. J Am Dent Assoc 1979;98:373.

6.  Thomson-Neal DM, Evans GH, Meffert RM, Davenport WD. An SEM evaluation of various prophylactic modalities on different implants. Int J Periodont Rest Dent 1989;9:301–311.

# 11

# Complications and Failure

*Philip Worthington*

Definitions of success and failure with oral implants have evolved over the years. It is now generally accepted that in order to be regarded as successful, an endosseous implant must do more than remain present in the jaw.[1] It must also demonstrate clinical immobility under load-bearing conditions, and it should be free from associated symptoms such as discomfort, pain, and tenderness. There should be no impairment of function of adjacent structures, such as the inferior alveolar nerve and its mental branch. There should be no progressive, continuing radiolucency surrounding the implant, and loss of crestal bone height should be minimal.

When failures occur they are usually, but not always, attributable to deviation from the procedures outlined in this text: patient selection may have been imprudent, planning may have been incomplete, consultation between clinicians may have been inadequate, or technique during the surgical, prosthetic and laboratory phases of treatment may have been faulty.

Osseointegration may fail to develop, or having developed, may later be lost. The causes of failed osseointegration are not always known. In some instances, it may be a biological failure; the bone may be too avascular or perhaps inadequate in quantity, quality, and density. It may be an iatrogenic failure; the bone may have been

## Success and Failure

overheated during implant site preparation. Osseointegration may be subsequently lost due to over-loading, perhaps due to poor prosthetic design, casting inaccuracy, or a patient's parafunctional habits.

## Endosseous Implants: Criteria of Success

- Clinical immobility
- Ability to bear load
- No associated symptoms
- No damage to adjacent structures
- No progressive peri-implant radiolucency
- Minimal loss of crestal bone height

## Indications of Failure

An implant that is persistently tender or that the patient says "just does not feel right" should be checked for failed osseointegration.

Mobility of an endosseous implant is a clear sign of failure, and such an implant should be removed. The clinician must distinguish, however, between the mobility of an incompletely attached abutment and the mobility of the underlying implant itself.

The development of a peri-implant radiolucent line on a radiograph is not usually an early sign of failure, but when present it indicates that the bone has receded from the implant surface and that the intervening space has been occupied by granulation tissue or a fibrous tissue sheath. This indicates incomplete osseointegration and probable implant failure.

When an individual implant fails, the clinician should remove it and possibly allow the site to heal completely before considering placement of a new implant. Under special circumstances, the implant site may be cleaned of granulation and fibrous tissue and an implant of greater diameter immediately placed.

# Complications

Complications may result from biological, iatrogenic, or mechanical factors. Biological factors tending to produce complications include bone of poor-quality or inadequate volume, smoking, and previous irradiation or immuno-suppression. Iatrogenic factors include inappropriate case selection, faulty planning, deviation from recommended surgical protocol, and prosthodontic overloading due to poor design. Mechanical factors include overly forceful manipulation and patient para-functional habits, such as bruxism.

## Complications Associated with Implant Placement

Faulty placement may take several forms. Implants may be placed too close together, so that it is difficult to attach the abutments or keep the intervening mucosa healthy. They may be placed too far to the labial or buccal aspect of the jaw, which may result in exposure of the implant as the site is enlarged (Fig 11-1). This may be remedied by the use of bone grafts or guided tissue regeneration to build up tissue volume. Similarly, implants placed too far lingually may suffer because of the thin, vulnerable, and mobile mucosa of the floor of the mouth. Faulty angulation of implants may be avoided by care in planning and by the use of surgical templates and guides, and may sometimes be remedied by the use of angulated abutments.

Excessive countersinking at the mouth of the implant site is to be avoided, especially in the posterior mandible, where internal support for the implant may be lacking due to the loosely textured trabecular bone.

A damaged, eccentric, or badly handled drill may result in an ovoid, rather than circular, implant site cross-section. The implant-bone contact is thus diminished, lessening the likelihood of successful osseointegration.

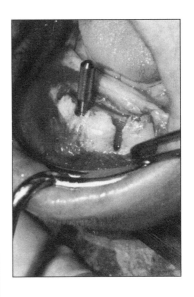

**Fig 11-1**  Labial placement of this implant resulted in exposure of the threads on the labial aspect. Had a template been used, this error might have been avoided.

When bone is overheated during the preparation of the implant site, bone cells in the immediate vicinity of the interface may not survive. The bone may die back from the implant surface and be replaced by less-differentiated scar tissue, making failure more likely. The use of sharp drills with intermittent and gentle pressure, drills of incremental sizes, copious coolant irrigation, and strictly controlled rotational drill speeds will minimize the risk of overheating.

Dehiscence of the incision may occur if there is premature loading of the recently operated site (eg, the premature wearing of a denture) or if the denture is inadequately relieved and cushioned over the implant sites. Breakdown of the wound is particularly likely if there has been previous irradiation (Fig 11-2) or surgery (such as a visor osteotomy or the placement and removal of a subperiosteal implant) in the implant area. These factors all tend to impair the blood supply of the area.

## Complications Associated with Abutment Connection

It is sometimes difficult to judge with accuracy the desirable height of the abutments when they are placed. One may need to change the abutments later, or use temporary healing abutments until the peri-implant soft tissues have stabilized.

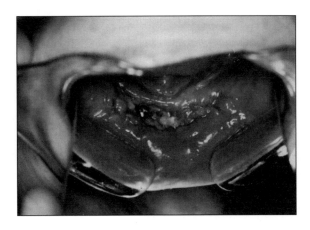

**Fig 11-2**  Dehiscence of the incision used for implant placement. In this instance this was attributed to previous irradiation of the area during treatment of an oral carcinoma.

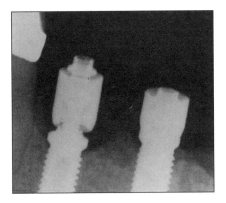

**Fig 11-3**  Note that one of the abutments in this radiograph is incompletely seated. This may lead to inflammatory problems and possible fistula formation. It should be corrected before treatment continues.

The abutment cylinder must be accurately seated on the implant. Many systems have interlocking hexagonal projections and recesses, and if the abutment cylinder is incompletely seated one may anticipate soft tissue hyperplasia, infection, and possible fistula formation (Fig 11-3).

Cover screws used to cover the ends of the implants during the bone healing phase sometimes require a hexagonal-head screwdriver. When the adjacent bone grips the cover screw very tightly, the tip of the screwdriver may fracture, leaving the broken segment in the cover screw. This broken part must then be removed.

## Complications Associated with Restoration and Maintenance

Abutment screws may loosen while the prosthetic device is being constructed; they must be checked periodically for tightness.

A prosthesis base that does not fit absolutely passively will cause unequal distribution of forces and may lead to serious problems. Complications include breakage of the abutment or retention screws and fracture of the cast base (Fig 11-4). Acrylic material used to provide the occlusal surface of the prosthesis may split and break off if it is not thick enough. Defective oral hygiene, particularly in association with mobile peri-implant mucosa, tends to produce gingivitis and gingival hyperplasia.

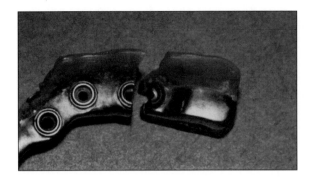

**Fig 11-4** Fracture of the whole prosthesis including the metal baseplate. The cross-sectional design of the baseplate casting is important, as is the length of the cantilever extension.

If there is a gap between the base plate and the alveolar crest of a maxillary implant-supported prosthesis, there may be an initial problem with air escaping during speech. This can be corrected in the short term by the wearing of a removable dam in the form of a gingival veneer. Usually, the patient undergoes a process of adaptation, after which the dam is not necessary.

## Serious Complications

The placement of dental implants, like other oral surgical procedures, carries a small risk of serious complications, including fatality. Death from air embolism has resulted from the mistaken use of a coolant spray of compressed air and water used with internally irrigated drills.[2] This misguided practice has also caused serious surgical emphysema. Such tragedies are avoidable. Practitioners should not deviate from the manufacturers' recommendations regarding the use of equipment.

Life-threatening hemorrhage has been reported due to instrumental perforation of the lingual cortex of the mandible during implant site preparation, with damage to small vessels in the adjacent floor of the mouth.[3,4] Bleeding may then progress into the soft tissues of the floor of the mouth, causing a threat to the patient's airway and necessitating emergency surgical treatment. Careful surgery, exploration of lingual concavities at operation, and postoperative patient supervision are needed to prevent this complication.

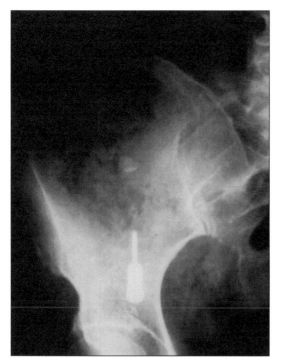

**Fig 11-5**  Radiograph shows a small screw-driver lodged in the patient's pelvis; its progress was arrested at the ileo-cecal junction. The instrument was later removed successfully by fiber optic colonoscopy.

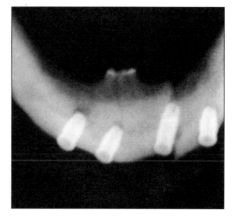

**Fig 11-6**  Fracture of the mandible through the site of an endosseous cylinder implant, shown on a radiograph.

Many implant components are small, as are the instruments involved. When coated with saliva, a component may escape from the clinician's grip and fall into the oropharynx, where reflex swallowing may take the item out of sight almost immediately. This is a particular risk with a recumbent patient (Fig 11-5). The item may thus be ingested, or even worse, inhaled. If this should happen, the patient should be immediately placed in a head-down position and an attempt made to recover the lost component. If it has gone too far, the patient should be transported to a hospital in a head-low position so that the appropriate endoscopy can be carried out.

Fracture of the atrophic mandible has been reported in several instances and certainly must have occurred in many unreported cases (Fig 11-6).[5] This emphasizes the

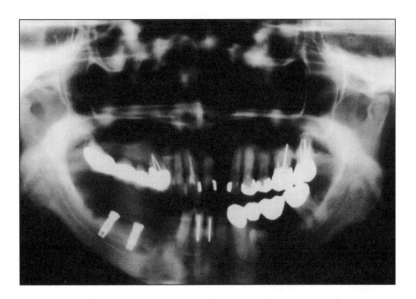

**Fig 11-7a**   Panoramic radiograph indicating probable intrusion of implants into inferior alveolar nerve canal.

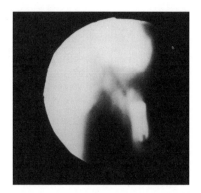

**Fig 11-7b**   This tomogram confirms the penetration of an endosseous implant into the inferior alveolar canal. This resulted in loss of sensation in the mental nerve territory.

need for great care in patient evaluation, surgery, and aftercare. Patients with an atrophic mandible must be warned to take great care in the postoperative period. Treatment of a fractured atrophic mandible is never easy, but when the jawbone contains several recently placed, expensive implants occupying space that might otherwise be used for plates and screws, the situation is even more critical.

Damage to the inferior alveolar nerve due to misplaced implants has been reported (Fig 11-7a and b). This indicates the need for detailed planning, including, in some cases, presurgical specialized radiographic assessment by CT scans.

## Minimizing Complications

All implant systems have their history of complications.[6,7] These can usually be avoided by attention to detail throughout the whole period of patient care, from patient selection and treatment planning to the clinical and maintenance phases. Many complications can be avoided with thorough planning and attentive treatment. Careful follow-up often provides early detection of incipient complications. With reputable implant systems, the problems and complications that do occur are usually due to deviation from recommended protocols, and should diminish in frequency as the clinician gains experience. Complications deserve our most serious attention, not merely because of their effects on patients, but because the reputation of implant dentistry as a whole is at stake. Restorative dentists need to exercise the greatest care throughout the entire treatment period; small errors in planning or technique may produce greatly magnified effects.

# References

1.  Albrektsson T, Zarb GA, Worthington P, Eriksson AR. The long term efficacy of currently used dental implants: A review and proposed criteria of success. Int J Oral Maxillofac Implants 1986;1:11–25.

2.  Davies JM, Campbell LA. Fatal air embolism during dental implant surgery: Report of three cases. Can J Anaesth 1990;37:112–121.

3.  Mason ME, Triplett, RG, Alfonso WF. Life-threatening hemorrhage from placement of a dental implant. J Oral Maxillofac Surg 1990;48:201–204.

4.  Laboda G. Life-threatening hemorrhage after the placement of an endosseous implant: Report of a case. J Am Dent Assoc 1990;121: 599–600.

5.  Mason ME, Triplett RG, van Sickels JE, Parel SM. Mandibular fractures through endosseous cylinder implants: Report of cases and review. J Oral and Maxillofac Surg 1990;8:311–317.

6.  Worthington P, Bolender CL, Taylor TD. The Swedish system of osseointegrated implants: Problems and complications encountered during a 4-year trial period. Int J Oral Maxillofac Implants 1987;2:77–84.

7.  Worthington P. Problems and complications with osseointegrated implants. In: Worthington P, Brånemark P-I (eds). Advanced Osseointegration Surgery: Applications in the Maxillofacial Region. Chicago: Quintessence, 1992:386–396.

# Conclusion

Osseointegration has now been applied in clinical practice since 1965. We know from extensive research and clinical trials that it works; this has been confirmed by multicenter trials in countries around the world. It succeeds given certain conditions, which include prudent patient selection, the use of biocompatible materials, meticulous adherence to the recommended surgical protocol, skillful prosthetic management, and long-term maintenance.

There is no denying that the surgical and prosthetic stages are highly technique-sensitive. Small variations in the execution of the practical steps can result in profound changes in the outcome.

Osseointegrated reconstruction demands respect for biology. The body's wound-healing processes must be harnessed to achieve osseointegration and conditions of overloading must be avoided in order not to destroy osseointegration.

This biological phenomenon has found a wide range of applications in orthopedic surgery and in craniofacial reconstruction, as well as in oral rehabilitation, where clinical application began. All over the world, thousands of dental patients have derived from osseointegration lasting benefits of a degree previously unimaginable.